PRAISE FOR DEEPAK CHOPRA

"Deepak Chopra is being hailed as a modern-day Hippocrates for his novel approach of combining ancient healing traditions with modern research."

> Irv Kupcinet,
> *Chicago Sun-Times*

"We can't help wishing he lived close enough to make house calls."

> Judith Hooper,
> *The New York Times Book Review*

"Dr. Chopra's writing has great beauty, great power, great delight, and much common sense."

> Courtney Johnson, author of
> *Henry James and the Evolution of Consciousness*

"Dr. Chopra presents us with information that can help us live long, healthy lives."

> Bernie Siegel, M.D., author of
> *Love, Medicine and Miracles*

DEEPAK CHOPRA, M.D.

PERFECT

WEIGHT

the complete mind/body program

for achieving and maintaining

your ideal weight

Crown Trade Paperbacks/New York

Published by Crown Trade Paperbacks, 201 East 50th Street, New York, New York 10022. Member of the Crown Publishing Group.

Originally published in hardcover by Harmony Books, a division of Crown Publishers, Inc., in 1994.

Random House, Inc. New York, Toronto, London, Sydney, Auckland

Portions of this book were originally published on audiocassette by Quantum Publications as part of the Perfect Health Series in 1991.

CROWN TRADE PAPERBACKS and colophon are trademarks of Crown Publishers, Inc.

Printed in the United States of America
Library of Congress Cataloging-in-Publication Data
Chopra, Deepak.
    Perfect weight : The complete mind/body program for achieving and maintaining your ideal weight / Deepak Chopra.
        p.   cm.
1. Reducing.   2. Medicine, Ayurvedic.   3. Mind and body.
I. Title.
RM222.2.C48   1994
613.2'5—dc20
94-19242
CIP

ISBN 0-517-88458-5
10 9 8 7 6 5 4 3 2 1

First Paperback Edition

CONTENTS

INTRODUCTION

Perfect Weight is not an ordinary weight control program. It's unique in many respects, but the fundamental difference between this book and other, more conventional approaches can be expressed quite simply. Instead of beginning with the assumption that there's something wrong with you that needs to be corrected, our starting point here is the idea that there's nothing essentially wrong with you at all. On the contrary, this program is based on the fact that you are inherently *perfect* ... and, even more important, you're absolutely *unique*.

Your ideal weight, therefore, cannot be expressed as a three-digit number on a chart mass-produced by an insurance company. The perfect weight for you is much more subjective. When you feel healthy, energetic, physically attractive, and comfortable with your body, then and only then are you at your ideal weight. You are the sole person who can determine this, and your own opinion is the only one that truly matters.

If you've been trying hard to live up to an artificial, media-generated notion of what the human body should look like, it's easy to forget that powerful forces of nature worked for millions of years to create you exactly as you are. Your body is a miracle of biological engineering. The underlying flawlessness of your body is always present, and grasping this fact is the first, all-important step toward genuine good health. Thus, despite what many authorities would have you believe, there's no need to create a "new you" in order to solve a weight problem, or for that matter, any other health problem. The real solution lies, quite simply, in recovering the perfect physiology that nature has already given you. And it's easier than you might think.

I recognize, of course, that all this may sound rather abstract. Right now you may not feel you're perfect. You may not be feeling good about yourself at all. There's an excellent chance you've tried one or more of the scores of weight control methods readily available at any given time. Many of these require you to carefully monitor the number of calories you consume. Others demand limited fat consumption, vigorous exercise, or a combination of the two. If you've tried such programs, the chances are that you did indeed lose weight, and perhaps very quickly at first. But there's also an overwhelming probability that you gained back all the weight you lost, and more, within twelve to eighteen months. Unfortunately, research indicates that the overall effects of losing and regaining weight are probably worse than those of being overweight in the first place.

Calorie counting, depriving yourself of foods you enjoy, and extreme physical exertion have no place in this book. Instead, you'll find simple, natural principles for balancing the mind and body. By learning to listen to your inner intelligence, you'll be able to restore the natural rhythms of your physiology and regain the unique perfection you were born with.

Let me once again emphasize the word *unique*. The combination of biological, emotional, and spiritual elements comprising your mind/body system is absolutely singular and cannot be defined by graphs, charts, or tables. Leaf through the pages of this book—you'll see no columns of numbers. Although my experience with literally thousands of patients over the years has enabled me to recognize certain norms based on height and weight, these are simply clinical observations; they're certainly not ideals held up with the intention of regulating behavior. While it may be true that many men who are five feet eight inches tall can feel healthy and energetic at a weight of 154 pounds, I would not prescribe this weight as "best" for all males of that height. To do so would simply be unrealistic, based on what I know about variations in the human physiology.

To help you identify the characteristics of your physiology, *Perfect Weight* includes a body-type questionnaire based on the traditional Indian science of health known as Ayurveda. By completing this questionnaire, and by becoming familiar with Ayurveda's astonishingly perceptive descriptions of the body and its variations, you can instantly gain access to five thousand years of wisdom about human health. With this as a starting point, you'll be able to recognize—perhaps for the first time—the real needs and rhythms of your body. You'll learn to see where, perhaps, you've broken with those rhythms and how to restore them. You'll gain the power to achieve *your* ideal weight without the physical pain, emotional stress, and eventual disappointment that are built into virtually all other weight control methods.

The fact is, once you've learned to live in accord with your biological needs instead of fighting against them, proper weight is literally achieved by itself. Cravings for unhealthy foods disappear. The loss of self-esteem that accompanies overweight is replaced by a sense of mental and physical well-being. Lack of energy and sedentary habits give way to enthusiasm for life and an eagerness to take part in it. To think of these natural processes in terms of struggle, as most diet programs do, will come to seem almost ludicrous. Grass, after all, doesn't "struggle" to grow, fish don't "struggle" to swim, and the Earth doesn't "struggle" its way around the sun!

I urge you to put the ideas and techniques of this book to work in your life as soon as possible, because the benefits of achieving and maintaining your ideal weight can be far-reaching indeed. This is especially true if you've tried other weight control methods and have been disappointed with the results. By regaining balance in this very significant area of your life, and by enjoying the sense of health and well-being that comes with it, you'll take an important, inspiring step toward fulfilling the truly unlimited potential that nature intends for you.

PERFECT
WEIGHT

UNDERSTANDING

THE TRUE NATURE OF YOUR

MIND AND BODY

Americans are extremely worried about the problem of overweight. For some of us, in my opinion, there's good reason for that concern, and for others there's not. But even when someone has valid concerns about his or her weight, the actions taken as a result are often ineffective and even dangerous to health. This confusing state of affairs has been documented many times with regard to crash diets, strenuous exercise regimes, and eating disorders such as anorexia and bulimia. The whole issue of weight control has become a muddle of contradictory evidence and constantly changing directives that has left us confused and perhaps somewhat fatalistic about the possibilities for positive change.

One of the primary goals of this book is to simplify the issues of weight control so that you can make intelligent decisions about how to achieve the weight you want, or how to feel more comfortable with the weight you have. To begin, let's look at some of the very few hard and fast truths that have emerged from all the concern with weight.

First, dieting—in the traditional sense of restricting food intake—almost always works in the short term and almost never works in the long term. You can pick virtually any of the dozens of commercially available diet plans, stick to it for a few months, and lose weight. But the lost weight, and probably even more, will come back over time. This has been the experience of virtually everyone who has undertaken serious dieting.

Second, while there are genuine health risks associated with overweight, there are also health risks related to weight loss— and the yo-yo effect that follows dieting may be the most dangerous of all. There is strong research evidence that bouncing up or down in weight poses significant health risks. In one study, men whose weight dropped by more than eleven pounds over a decade had a significantly higher mortality rate than those whose weight remained stable. And while research into the eating habits of extremely long-lived individuals has not isolated any particular food or dietary program that accounts for their longevity, there is evidence that such people definitely maintain a constant, consistent weight throughout their adult lives.

Last, the emotional effects of weight control should be given very serious consideration. I think this is the lesson of a remarkable study carried out in Finland, where heart attack rates are among the highest in the world. Twelve hundred business executives who were assumed to be at high risk for cardiac disease because of obesity, hypertension, high cholesterol levels, or heavy smoking were asked to follow a strict regimen of low-fat diet, medical exams, and access to information about potential risks. Meanwhile, another group of similarly high-risk individuals was left to do whatever they liked. Amazingly, after five years, death rates turned out to be much higher for the strictly monitored group. The only explanation seems to be that the stress and worry created by following an unfamiliar "healthy" lifestyle more than canceled any benefits of the lifestyle itself.

Issues of weight and health, as you can see, are more complex than simply consuming fewer calories or switching from butter to margarine. As long as clinical obesity is not present—defined as being 25 percent above normal weight for your height—what you should weigh is really a more subjective matter than has been widely recognized. Perhaps the most important consideration should be your ability to feel in control of your body. If you feel your weight is something that's just happened to you, like a broken leg, you're certainly justified in changing that situation. On the other hand, if you're comfortable with your current proportions (and you're not obese), you shouldn't let anyone else's views displace your own. In short, you may already be at your ideal weight. But if you're not, this book will show you how to identify that ideal goal, how to reach it without emotional stress or physical pain, and how to maintain it for many years to come.

A VERY BRIEF HISTORY

Let's look for a moment at the historical events that led to our present obsession with body weight.

In 1876, one hundred years after the signing of the Declaration of Independence, the head of an American middle-class family could be expected to eat a "good" breakfast. This might include steak, bacon and eggs, fried potatoes, pancakes, sausage, porridge, doughnuts, and fruit—all at one sitting.

That seems excessive, doesn't it? Even if it had been the consumption of an entire day, it would be out of line with most current recommendations about diet. As a single meal, it seems positively gluttonous!

But consider this: After eating such a breakfast, a man would most likely begin a twelve- to fourteen-hour workday on a farm or in some form of heavy industry such as steel-making or railroads. Further, standards for judging a healthy and attractive appearance were very different. In a time when the gaunt face of tuberculosis was widespread, particularly among the poor, fat was a sign of financial prosperity and physical well-being. A hundred years ago many widely admired Americans were grossly overweight, at least by today's criteria. Just one example is William Howard Taft, who in the early years of the twentieth century was both U.S. president and chief justice of the Supreme Court; he weighed more than 300 pounds and often needed help to get out of the bathtub.

Even in the nineteenth century, however, voices could be heard condemning extravagant eating and its effects on the body. The Kellogg and Post cereal companies began as purveyors of health food. Shredded wheat was invented in 1892 by a Denver vegetarian named Henry Perky.

Competing attitudes toward food, eating, and weight are still with us, perhaps more strongly than ever. But some significant changes have taken place to make the struggle even more intense. For one thing, when refrigerators became available to the public around the time of World War I, with them came the ready availability of such perishable items as butter, cream, and even ice cream—to say nothing of more recent innovations such as soft drinks, chocolate syrup, and high-fat frozen foods. Meanwhile, daily life has been getting easier—at least in terms of physical labor. The backbreaking work that used to offset a breakfast of steak and eggs has been replaced by tapping computer keys and holding a telephone.

At the beginning of the twentieth century, human labor

accounted for a large part of the energy needed to produce society's goods and services. Today, when physical labor directly accounts for almost none of our goods and services, and we have instant access to a wide range of tempting but very fattening foods, a greater number of people than ever before meets the medical standard for obesity. But a tremendous amount of guilt has come with all that eating, and also widespread (though often futile) efforts to change. Surveys reveal that during any given year one-half of the American population starts a diet for weight reduction; approximately 50 million Americans are on a diet at any one time; 75 percent of American women think they should lose weight; Americans spend more than $30 billion each year in efforts to lose weight or at least prevent weight gain. Yet the average woman today weighs five to six pounds more than she did twenty years ago, and the weight of Americans in general is going up.

What is responsible for this contradictory behavior? Why are people gaining weight, sometimes to the point where their health is threatened, despite their attempts to change? Why do 98 percent of all weight-loss programs fail? To answer these questions you need to grasp certain remarkable ideas about your body and how it functions.

I want to introduce to you the concept of the quantum mechanical body/mind. Once you understand the true character of the body and the true nature of the mind, once you see them and know them as they really are, this knowledge will by itself have a dramatic effect on how you behave with regard to your weight. Indeed, it can have an important effect on how you perceive your life as a whole.

The concept of the human body that most of us accept is actually based on a superstition. Specifically, it's based on the superstition of materialism.

By *materialism* I'm referring to the idea that just because something looks the way it does, that's the way it must truly be. To a certain extent, of course, everyone must be a materialist in order to get through the day. But in a very basic sense materialism does not express what we now know about the true nature of reality. Some instances of this are quite obvious: The Earth looks flat, but we know it's round; we think the ground we are standing on is perfectly stationary, yet we know it's spinning at dizzying speeds as it hurtles through outer space at thousands of miles per hour. Other examples of the limits of materialism, as you'll see in a moment, are more subtle, but the point remains the same. We cannot fully trust our senses.

Even though our senses tell us that the body is a solid, frozen, anatomical structure, fixed in space and time, this is not really the case. The truth is that our bodies are rivers of intelligence, information, and energy—constantly renewing themselves in every second of their existence. Just as you cannot step into exactly the same river twice, you cannot inhabit the same flesh and bones for even a fraction of a second, because in every instant you're literally creating a new body.

You change your body more effortlessly, more spontaneously, and more expeditiously than you can change your clothes. In fact, right now, this very second, the body that you're using to read this book is not the same one you started out with a few minutes ago.

In Ayurveda (the Sanskrit word meaning "the science of life"), the system of traditional Indian medicine on which this book is based, the human body is defined as a fluctuation of energy and information in a larger field of energy and information. The body is not so much a "thing" as it is a *process*. Therefore we will focus not on the molecules that make up your body but on the functioning—the shifting and changing and flowing—of those processes that comprise your body. And for our present purposes, of course, the most important functions are eating, breathing, digestion, metabolism, elimination, and a very fundamental activity known as the movement of consciousness, which in fact is the foundation of all the others.

Let's take just one example: the act of breathing. With every breath, you inhale 10^{22} atoms from the universe. This astronomical volume of raw material enters your body from your environment and quickly becomes the cells of your heart, bones, kidneys, and liver. Then, with every exhaled breath, you release the same number of atoms from every part of your body. You're literally *breathing out* bits and pieces of your heart and kidneys.

So, technically speaking, we're sharing our organs with other people all the time—and not only with our contemporaries but with everyone who ever lived. Based on mathematical computations of radioactive isotopes, it can be shown without a shadow of doubt that right now, in your physical body, you have a million atoms that were once in the body of Jesus or the Buddha or Genghis Khan or Leonardo da Vinci or Michelangelo. Just in the last three weeks a quadrillion atoms—which is 10 followed by fifteen zeroes—have gone through your body that have also passed through the bodies of every other living species on this planet.

In less than one year, 98 percent of all the atoms in your body are replaced completely. This includes even the DNA, which holds memories of millions of years of evolutionary time. The actual raw material of your DNA—the carbon, hydrogen, nitrogen, and oxygen—comes and goes like migratory birds every six weeks.

In sum, you are literally changing your body as effortlessly as you change your clothes, with an almost infinite number of atoms literally coming and going in the twinkling of an eye. The American poet Walt Whitman wrote: "Every atom belonging to you as well belongs to me." This may have been meant as a metaphor, but it is the literal truth.

YOUR BODY AS IT REALLY IS

Although what you've just read may seem remarkable, it's really only the beginning. What *are* these atoms that are ceaselessly flowing in and out of your body?

Suppose you went to a physicist and asked: "What is the essential nature of this basic unit of matter that makes up the flesh and bones of my body?" You would learn that an atom is made up of particles—but the particles are not really material objects; imagining that they are is another superstition. Rather, the particles are fluctuations of energy and information in a void of energy and information. The essential raw material of the body turns out to be *nonmaterial*.

If you could see the body as it really is, you'd see a huge void with a few scattered dots and spots and some random electrical discharges. In fact, 99.999996 percent of the body is mostly empty space. And if you could truly understand the .000004 percent of the body that appears to be solid matter, you would realize that it's also empty space, every bit of it. But at the same time, it is *intelligence*. This nonmaterial quality of information that regulates, constructs, governs, and actually becomes the body. And that same intelligence of inner space is part of a continuum with outer space!

Nature goes to the same source for material to create a galaxy, a rain forest, or a human body as it goes to create a thought. This is fundamental to the approach of this book, in which you'll see that the fluctuations in consciousness that we call thoughts and feelings are actually a reflection of the underlying intelligence that structures the mind/body system. By understanding the nature of that intelligence and allowing it to take dynamic form, you can transform your body into its ideal state. Because the truth is that there's a joyful, healthy, perfect body within you just waiting to be unfolded.

METABOLISM AND SELF-REFERRAL

Your body's metabolism, which governs how food is consumed and converted into energy, operates under what we might call both *macro* and *micro* influences. The macro, or larger, influence is that profound intelligence that we have been discussing, which animates the entire universe. At the same time, our emotions, feelings, desires, and thought processes constantly modulate and change our metabolic profile, and this is what I mean by the "micro" influence. Certain emotions speed up your metabolism, and other emotions slow it down. Some emotions cause excessive secretion of acid in the stomach, while others have an opposite effect. Whatever is going on in that network of intelligence is constantly expressing itself as these various metabolic processes.

In order to direct your personal emotions, as well as the larger, univeral intelligence, toward perfect health, I would like you to begin a process that is known in Ayurveda as *self-referral*. In our society self-referral is, unfortunately, very uncommon. It simply means looking within yourself and your internal value system in order to influence your thoughts or actions. The alternative to self-referral is object-referral, whereby people respond to external cues that govern their behavior.

Self-referral occurs when you direct your attention to follow internal cues. These internal cues are messages of comfort and discomfort that are emitted by our physiology in order to allow us to be perfectly healthy. You see, nature, in its infinite wisdom, really gives us only two messages: a sense of comfort and a sense of discomfort. When you're feeling perfectly comfortable in every way—physically, emotionally, and spiritually—then you're heading in the right direction. I call this *the state of spontaneous right action*, because the perfect response is present in your body/mind for every situation just as it occurs. The absolutely ideal reaction to every occurrence in your life is readily available to your body/mind when you are in the state of spontaneous right action. This is due to the wisdom of nature, which has endowed not only your physical body but the entire universe with this inner intelligence.

In order to tap in to this inner intelligence, you need only use the process of attention—so let's start out with a specific assignment to help direct your attention to the inner intelligence of your body. This assignment will help you to identify and know more about your appetite and eating habits.

GETTING STARTED

The assignment is quite simple and can be expressed in just one sentence: *Eat whenever you're hungry, but when you're not hungry, don't eat.*

For two weeks I would like you to follow this instruction as closely as possible.

The wisdom of this may seem self-evident, but in fact most people eat without relation to hunger. They eat because of habit, or social influences, or the stresses of jobs and relationships—in other words, because of object-referral. These people look for external cues in order to initiate their behavior, whether it's eating or sleeping or working. If that's been your pattern, we're going to change it.

Remember: Hunger is simply a signal from your body's intelligence that it wishes to eat and is prepared for the proper metabolism of the food that is to be consumed. If hunger is not present, nutrition is not required at that time, and the body is not prepared to metabolize it.

Here's an analogy that I think will illustrate my point. If you were driving past a gas station and noticed that you were low on fuel, it would make perfect sense for you to pull into the station and fill your tank. But suppose that as you were driving past the station you looked at your gas gauge and saw that your tank was full. If you *still* pulled into the station and attempted to put gas into your tank, this would not be productive behavior. It would provide no benefit to your car, and soon it would start to make a mess. Worst of all, even you would know that it was not in your best interests. Yet this is what takes place when you eat when you're not hungry.

Of course, the experience of eating is much more emotionally charged and satisfying than that of putting gas in a car. Food can be a friend when you're lonely. Preparing food can give you a sense of control when other areas of your life seem unmanageable. Going to the store and buying food can evoke a feeling of abundance that compensates for painful emptiness. Determining whether you're truly hungry is complicated, so to help you carry out the assignment of eating only when you're hungry, I've created a technique to help you become aware of your actual hunger level and the appropriate way to satisfy it.

This Satisfaction Meter will help you understand more about eating in accord with your hunger. Unlike the gas tank of a car, the stomach requires some room to allow proper digestion. If there is no room left in the stomach, you'll experience discomfort, distention, heaviness, and improper digestion; consistently eating until the stomach is entirely full produces metabolic toxins for the physiology and ultimately leads to obesity.

Let's look at the different levels on the Satisfaction Meter and what they mean.

Level 0 to 1. As digestion takes place, there comes a point at which you sense no remnant of food in your stomach from the previous meal. Your stomach seems empty, and you have the feeling of hunger. At this level, you should always eat. You're not starving, but there is a definite and genuine need that requires satisfaction.

SATISFACTION METER

How to use your **Satisfaction Meter:**
1. Whenever you are ready to eat, place your hand on your stomach, as a way of putting attention on that area of the body.
2. Then use the following scale to assess your hunger level:

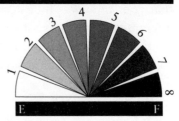

Level 0–1	Your stomach is completely empty—you cannot feel the presence of food in your system from the previous meal. At the same time, there is a sensation of hunger. This is the point at which you should start eating.
Levels 2, 3, 4	This is how you feel when you are eating comfortably, or after you've just eaten and are comfortably digesting the food. You do not feel hunger at these levels.
Level 5	As you are eating, you start to feel satisfied.
Level 6	This is the point of maximum comfort. You feel completely satisfied—there is neither a sensation of hunger nor any discomfort from overeating. This is the level at which you should stop eating.

AVOID THESE LEVELS

Levels 7 and 8	You have gone beyond the level of comfort. After eating there is a sensation of discomfort, such as heaviness, dullness, and distension of the abdomen.
Level F	You can't eat another bite. Your stomach is full to the point of distension and discomfort, like some people feel after eating Thanksgiving dinner.
Level E	Your stomach is uncomfortably empty. You are starving. **It is important to eat before you reach this level.**

3. For the next two weeks, start eating only if you are in the 0 to 1 range. This may mean eating meals at unusual times of day, or even not eating for prolonged periods of time. However, the entire process should be based on comfort. Always stop eating when you reach Level 6.

4. During these two weeks, use the **Daily Record of Hunger Levels** (next page) to record the time of day and your hunger level each time you eat. You should record not only meals but any snacks you eat.

DAILY RECORD OF HUNGER LEVELS

Directions: Each time you eat during the day, fill in the blanks indicating what time you ate, your hunger level before eating, and your hunger level after eating. Be sure to record your hunger level every time you eat, even if it is only a snack.

	Mon.	Tues.	Wed.	Thur.	Fri.	Sat.	Sun.
Time you ate							
Hunger level before eating							
Hunger level after eating							
Time you ate							
Hunger level before eating							
Hunger level after eating							
Time you ate							
Hunger level before eating							
Hunger level after eating							
Time you ate							
Hunger level before eating							
Hunger level after eating							
Time you ate							
Hunger level before eating							
Hunger level after eating							
Time you ate							
Hunger level before eating							
Hunger level after eating							
Time you ate							
Hunger level before eating							
Hunger level after eating							

Levels 2, 3, and 4. This range describes how you feel as you're comfortably continuing to eat, or later, after you've eaten, when the food is being comfortably digested. If you focus on it, you can definitely sense the presence of food in your stomach. There is no sensation of hunger associated with these levels.

Level 5. You start to feel satisfied.

Level 6. This is the point of maximum comfort. This is where you should stop eating.

Levels 7 and 8. The stomach is completely and uncomfortably full.

Level F. You can't possibly eat another bite. Even the thought of food makes you feel sick. Your stomach feels distended, as if you'd just had Thanksgiving dinner. Level F, of course, should be avoided.

Level E. The stomach is uncomfortably empty, and there's a starving sensation. Like being overly full, Level E is a deviation from the self-referral path of comfort. You should eat before you get to this level.

With practice, you'll be able to identify your level of satisfaction at any given moment. Try placing your hand over your stomach several times a day in order to direct your awareness to that area of your body. This is what I call the *value of attention,* and it has applications in all areas of your life.

Once you've assessed the true level of your hunger, remember that Ayurveda says you should eat to about three-fourths of your stomach's capacity, but not beyond that. This, of course, is the definition of level 6 on your Satisfaction Meter. Eating beyond this point causes discomfort, either at once or within an hour or two after the meal.

If you feel heavy, sleepy, or dull after a meal, you probably ate too much, but you can adjust next time. There's no need for guilt. Making mistakes is part of the learning process.

In carrying out your assignment of eating only when you're hungry, you may find yourself taking meals at unusual times of day. And sometimes you will eat very little, even for twenty-four hours or more. This is only because your biological rhythms are readjusting. If you're not eating, it shouldn't be because you're trying to diet but simply because you're not hungry. If you *are* hungry—that is, if you're at level 0 or 1 on the meter—go ahead and eat. Don't try to resist. But for the first two weeks of this program, you should not eat, regardless of the time, unless you are at level 0 or 1. You can be sure you're at this level when you cannot feel the presence of any food from a prior meal in your stomach and you feel a definite sensation of hunger.

Following this instruction for two weeks will give you time to become more aware of your body's inner signals. However, this is not a good routine to follow on a long-term basis. After the initial resetting of your body's inner intelligence, it is better to adjust your body's biological clock by taking lunch at the same time every day. For most people, this will happen quite naturally within about two weeks. You will find that you are hungry around lunchtime, especially if you eat only a light breakfast.

Ideally, ending your meals when you reach level 6 will become a lifelong habit. This is not dieting, it's simply paying attention to your body and its level of genuine satisfaction. Dieting implies strain, effort, and discomfort. This, in contrast, is a technique for ensuring *no discomfort.*

At the beginning of this chapter, when we took note of the almost universal concern regarding body weight, I suggested that the validity of this concern may vary from one individual to another. Now, using the terminology of self-referral and object-referral, let's analyze the basis of your concern. To help you do this, let me refer you to those very significant two words in the book's subtitle: *ideal weight.*

This phrase can be defined according to object-referral and to self-referral. It's very important for you to understand the difference and to realize which definition is motivating your actions.

A good example of the object-referral definition of ideal weight is provided by the tables insurance companies use to classify weight according to height. Versions of these often appear on public scales and in books or articles on dieting. These tables are meant to predict health and longevity as a result of weight. Whether the tables really perform this function is a subject beyond the scope of this book, but they definitely lead a large number of people to the conclusion that they're too heavy, and to feel bad about it as a result.

Another instance of an object-referral definition of ideal weight derives from examples set by exceedingly thin fashion models or celebrities, by the advertisements for diet programs and exercise machines, or by any one of a hundred other external influences that we are exposed to every day. When the phrase *ideal weight* is used in this book, these are *not* the definitions that are intended, and I hope they are not definitions that guide your decisions about your weight or health.

The self-referral definition of ideal weight comes from you, not from an insurance company or an advertising agency. It is the point at which you believe you will look and feel your best, based on a realistic assessment of yourself and your goals. This should not be the equivalent of saying you want to be an Olympic athlete or a world-renowned opera singer. Such notions will only set you up for defeat and disappointment. *Your ideal weight should be a self-referring, worthwhile, attainable goal.*

In order to better define your goal, answer the following questions in a paragraph or two on a separate sheet of paper, or just seriously consider them in your mind for a period of time. From time to time throughout this book, I'll suggest that you return to this list to see if your ideas have altered.

1. Why do you want your weight to change?
2. What do you want your weight to be?
3. Is there any reason you chose this number *except* your sincere belief that you would feel your best, emotionally and physically? If so, what would your ideal weight be if you were to eliminate those reasons?
4. At what age did you last weigh that amount?
5. Based on the inevitable changes that have taken place since then—in your age, your lifestyle, your responsibilities to work and to family—do you feel your answer to question 2 is self-referring, worthwhile, and attainable? *If so, that number represents your ideal weight.*

2

DISCOVERING YOUR

AYURVEDIC BODY TYPE

Ａs with all aspects of life, people respond individually to food, so a successful weight control program should be carefully designed to meet your individual needs. Ayurveda teaches that every health-related procedure—whether it's eating certain foods or following a particular exercise program—must be evaluated in terms of the constitution of the person using it.

This is in contrast to much of the practice of Western health care, in which the properties of various medicines are often more closely scrutinized than the characteristics of the individuals for whom those medicines are prescribed. But these essential elements of the patient and the treatment really should not be separated.

When a patient sees a Western physician for the first time he or she is usually asked to fill out a medical-history form; this is mostly to learn whether there have been any surgeries and to clarify what symptoms the patient is experiencing. Ayurveda, on the other hand, is concerned with information of a more basic kind. What is the *essential nature* of this person? What is the foundation of this person's body/mind system? Therefore Ayurveda teaches that anything a physician prescribes for you—or anything that you do for yourself—must be undertaken with an understanding of your individual makeup and the specific needs that derive from it.

In this chapter we'll discuss the physiological principles that make individual reactions such unique phenomena, and at the end of the chapter you'll fill out a questionnaire to determine your own Ayurvedic mind/body type.

This is vital information, for only by knowing your body type can you get in touch with your body's inner intelligence, which is the true source of everything that comprises your life. Because whether you're responding to food, the weather, a love note, or criticism from the boss, you're really acting in accord with a signal that is generated nowhere but within yourself.

Another difference between Ayurveda and contemporary Western medicine is that in the latter, a great deal of attention has been devoted to isolating differences among various diseases. This is very important information; it is extremely useful to know that there are three categories of hepatitis and five kinds of measles. But it's also very important to recognize the unique qualities of individual human beings, and this is an area in which Western health care has been less astute. This system really has no terminology for describing human similarities and differences in an organized way. But such a terminology is absolutely fundamental to Ayurveda, which recognizes the existence of constitutional types as the first step toward understanding health and illness.

Have you ever noticed that on a cool day some people are dressed in hats, scarves, and gloves, as if anticipating cold weather, while others are wearing short-sleeved shirts? Some people, after a quick lunch of a hot dog and french fries, are able to work well throughout the afternoon, while others require a completely different level of nutrition. After one cup of coffee some people get jittery, but others are completely unaffected. What is the basis of all these variations? It's not something that can be revealed by an X ray or a CAT scan, but it's very real nonetheless. Different shapes, sizes, personalities, and physiological characteristics define biochemical individuality, and Ayurveda has organized this information into a system of psychophysiological body types.

Your biochemical individuality expresses unique patterns of intelligence that exist within your body type. In Ayurveda, the word for body type is *prakriti*, a Sanskrit term that literally means "essential nature." Thus, the body type is like a blueprint outlining innate tendencies that have been built into every aspect of your mind/body system.

Learning about your Ayurvedic body type will give you useful information on how to reawaken your body's inner intelligence. You'll be able to identify which foods, activities, and medications will have the greatest benefit. Each of these is a personal message that your physiology interprets according to its unique characteristics of mind and body. But be aware that the distinction between these two elements has its limits: mind and body intersect. Every time there's an event in the mind, for example, there's a corresponding event in the body. At the junction point where thought becomes physical event, Ayurveda defines three governing agents. These are the *doshas*—quantum mechanical mind/body principles that govern the flow of intelligence throughout the physiology.

In simple terms, here's how the doshas express themselves: If you are of rather slender build and have very irregular eating habits, you might suddenly feel hungry at any time of the day. Similarly, your sleep patterns might be very unpredictable— sometimes you sleep for the first several hours after going to bed, but then you awaken and can't get back to sleep, so you get up and eat a sandwich. Based on this information, I would be able to identify which one of the three doshas was dominant in you. However, if you tell me that you live by your watch, particularly where meals are concerned, and that you become ravenously hungry if dinner is even thirty minutes late, I would recognize another dosha as being your dominant influence. And of course there are people who are neither noticeably regular nor irregular in their personal habits—people who might use a word such as *easygoing* to describe themselves. In them, a third dosha is dominant.

People are often amazed by the ability of Ayurvedic physicians to arrive at a deep understanding of their characteristics, both biological and psychological, based on just a few facts about their eating and sleeping habits. But there's nothing magical about it. Ayurveda (which you'll recall is the Sanskrit term meaning "the science of life") is the world's oldest system of health care. It is based on an understanding of the relationship between man and the rest of nature, and it was born long before that relationship became as obscure as it is today. Ayurveda is, quite literally, the wisdom of the ages. However, Ayurveda is not the only tradition that recognizes the existence of specific physiological categories. In medieval Europe there emerged a system of understanding individuals in terms of four "humors," which were derived from the natural elements of earth, air, fire, and water. The temperaments and behaviors of individuals were explained by an excess of a particular humor. Hamlet, for instance, is traditionally dressed in black throughout Shakespeare's play. To the seventeenth-century audience, this indicated an excess of the earth-related humor, which produces a melancholy disposition. As you shall see, there is an obvious analogy between this and Ayurvedic terminology. And even very experienced Western physicians, working within a frame of reference that would seem counter to any ancient system of "folk beliefs," have come intuitively to recognize physical and psychological characteristics that predispose individuals to conditions such as coronary disease and cancer. Dr. Paul Dudley White, for example, who was President Eisenhower's personal physician, observed that tall, slender individuals rarely suffer heart attacks, which are much more likely to strike people with shorter, broader physiques, particularly barrel-chested males. In short, no health care system or individual physician has a monopoly on wisdom, but the Ayurvedic method of categorizing people according to the influence of the three doshas is the most practical and comprehensive approach of which I am aware.

For our purposes here, that approach means simply that a weight control program may work very well for a certain individual but be quite ineffective for others who are constituted according to a fundamentally different mind/body system. Your body type, whose tendencies you inherited at birth, is the most natural guide to how you should eat, exercise, and make decisions in every area of your life.

The three doshas that comprise the Ayurvedic body types are *Vata*, *Pitta*, and *Kapha*. Although they control all the endless combinations of processes that comprise your being, each of the doshas is related to certain elements in nature as a whole. The doshas are literally everywhere—in the weather, in plants and animals, and most definitely in foods. Even the times of day and the seasons of the year have their doshas. These three elements connect you as an individual to the entire organization of the universe. The unity of nature intimately connects the large plan to the small one, which is your individual character. The better you understand these connections, the more rewarding your life will be.

Each of the three doshas has certain basic, well-defined functions:

• *Vata dosha*, which is related to air, controls all movement in the body: the movement of vocal cords as you speak, the movement of thought, the movement of your hands and feet, the movement of blood as it flows through your heart. Vata qualities are dry, cold, light, and, above all, changeability. When in balance, Vata maintains energy, motion, and respiration. Out of balance, it can bring about dehydration, coldness throughout the body, and emotional instability.

• *Pitta dosha*, which is related to fire, controls metabolism and digestion. In balance, Pitta properly regulates hunger, thirst, heat throughout the body, and the acuity of intelligence. But aggravated Pitta can bring on sensations of anger, frustration, and, most important for our purposes, extreme hunger.

• *Kapha dosha*, which derives from water and from earth, controls the structure of the body, even down to the cellular level. Kapha maintains strength and physical form through the bones, muscles, and tendons. When out of balance, it can cause congestive illnesses such as colds and flu, and it is principally responsible for conditions of overweight.

THE THREE DOSHAS

The Basic Functions	Their Qualities
VATA	
Governs bodily functions concerned with movement	Moving, quick, light, cold, minute, rough, dry; leads the other doshas
PITTA	
Governs bodily functions concerned with heat and metabolism	Hot, sharp, light, acidic, slightly oily
KAPHA	
Governs bodily functions concerned with structure and fluid balance	Heavy, oily, slow, cold, steady, solid, dull

TEN CONSTITUTIONAL TYPES

ONE-DOSHA TYPES

Vata	Pitta	Kapha

TWO-DOSHA TYPES

Vata-Pitta	Pitta-Kapha	Vata-Kapha
Pitta-Vata	Kapha-Pitta	Kapha-Vata

THREE-DOSHA TYPE

Vata-Pitta-Kapha

Although your body type expresses dominance by one of the doshas, or perhaps a combination of them, every cell in your body must contain all three doshas to remain alive. You need Vata (motion) to breathe, to circulate your blood, to pass food through your digestive tract, and to send nerve impulses between your brain and the rest of your body. You need Pitta (metabolism) to process food, air, and water through your entire system and to allow for proper intellectual functioning. And you must have Kapha (structure) to hold your cells together and to form connective tissue.

Although nature needs all three doshas to build and sustain a human body, each of us is constituted differently in terms of the amount of each dosha we contain. Only a small percentage of people are purely Vata, Pitta, or Kapha types. Each of us possesses a proportion of all three doshas. Often two doshas combine to dominate and therefore characterize an individual's physiology, and occasionally all three can be found in equal measure.

By knowing your body type, you can become aware of the dosha that is most prominent in your physiology. This will help you to create habits of diet, exercise, and daily routine that maintain ideal weight and promote perfect health. This is the essential nature you inherited. This is *who* you are and *what* you are.

Here are some brief descriptions of the traits and behaviors that characterize the three doshas.

VATA

Characteristics of Vata Type

- Light, thin build
- Performs activity quickly
- Irregular hunger and digestion
- Light, interrupted sleep; tendency toward insomnia
- Enthusiasm, vivaciousness, imagination
- Excitability, changing moods
- Quick to grasp new information, also quick to forget
- Tendency to worry
- Tendency to be constipated
- Tires easily, tendency to overexert
- Mental and physical energy comes in bursts

It is very Vata to
- Be hungry at any time of the day or night
- Love excitement and constant change
- Go to sleep at different times every night, skip meals, and keep irregular habits in general
- Digest food well one day and poorly the next
- Display bursts of emotion that are short-lived and quickly forgotten
- Walk quickly

Vata types have a light, thin build. They perform activity quickly. Rapid movement is a feature of their actions. They may have irregular hunger and digestion, and their sleep is often light and interrupted. When under stress they easily get insomnia. They tire easily and tend to overexert, and their mental and physical energy may come in bursts.

Usually, Vata types are enthusiastic, vivacious, and imaginative. But their emotions can change quickly, so under stress those characteristics may be transformed into anxiety. Usually Vata types are quick to grasp new information, but they are also quick to forget.

In general, Vata people are unpredictable and much less stereotyped than either Pittas or Kaphas. So it is very Vata to be hungry at any time of the day or night, to love excitement and constant change, to go to sleep at different times every night, to skip meals, and to keep irregular habits in general.

Since Vata goes out of balance more easily than the other doshas, it's important to create stability and regularity in your habits in order to keep Vata imbalance from occurring. Vata controls the impulses of the nervous system, and therefore impulsiveness can usually be traced to an imbalance in this dosha. If you eat whenever you get the urge, for instance, I would say that you have a great deal of Vata in your eating behavior. This kind of impulsive eating by Vata types is especially evident when they're under stress or when they feel threatened. "I seem to just stop eating," or, "It's as if nothing could possibly taste good to me," a Vata type might say. Or the impulsive behavior might go in a completely different direction. In extreme cases, when the Vata dosha becomes seriously unbalanced, any calories consumed are used up by nervous energy and chaotic activity. They're metabolized so rapidly that nothing gets stored as fat. This may seem appealing to a person who's overweight, but it's definitely not a healthy state of affairs. In deep stages of Vata imbalance, muscle tissues may begin to waste away.

With respect to eating habits, therefore, Vata types should take their meals on a regular schedule and should be sure to select a balanced variety of foods. Vatas should avoid cold foods and drinks, which will immediately unbalance the dosha. Heavy, hearty foods that have a settling and comforting effect should be emphasized, such as stews, breads, and warm desserts. Everything should be thoroughly cooked, and raw fruits and vegetables should make up only a small part of a Vata-balancing diet.

PITTA

Characteristics of Pitta Type

- Medium build
- Medium strength and endurance
- Sharp hunger and thirst, strong digestion
- Tendency to become angry or irritable under stress
- Fair or ruddy skin, often freckled
- Aversion to sun, hot weather
- Enterprising character, likes challenges
- Sharp intellect
- Precise, articulate speech
- Cannot skip meals
- Blond, light brown, or red hair (or reddish undertones)

It is very Pitta to
- Feel ravenous if dinner is half an hour late
- Live by your watch and resent having your time wasted
- Wake up at night feeling hot and thirsty
- Take command of a situation or feel that you should
- Learn from experience that others find you too demanding, sarcastic, or critical at times
- Have a determined stride when you walk

Pitta types are usually of medium build, with average levels of strength and endurance. They are fair in appearance, with ruddy, often freckled skin. They may have a strong aversion to sun and hot weather. Their hunger and thirst is felt very sharply. They have strong digestions and they hate to skip meals.

Pittas have a tendency to get angry under stress, but they're enterprising characters who like challenges. They have a sharp intellect and very precise, articulate speech. The basic theme of the Pitta type is intensity. Anyone who has bright red hair and a florid face contains a good deal of Pitta dosha, as does anyone who is ambitious, sharp-witted, outspoken, bold, argumentative, or jealous.

When in balance, Pitta types are warm and ardent in their emotions, and they can be very loving. A face glowing with happiness is very Pitta. It is also very Pitta to feel ravenously hungry if dinner is half an hour late, to live by your watch (generally an expensive one), and to resent having your time wasted. It is Pitta to wake up at night feeling hot and thirsty, and to take command of a situation or to feel that you should. Pitta types walk with a determined stride. They often learn that others find them too demanding and occasionally too sarcastic and critical.

Since they're convinced that their robust digestion can handle anything, Pitta types tend to overeat. When they've eaten too much and caused their prominent dosha to go out of balance, Pittas are prone to stomach and intestinal pain, heartburn, and even ulcers. Therefore Pitta types should eat moderately and not abuse their excellent digestion. They should avoid eating when angry or emotional and should try to take meals in relaxed settings that will create the proper mood. Eating outdoors amid the beauty of nature is especially good for Pitta types. Unlike Vata types, Pittas benefit from cold drinks and salads. Spicy or very hot food should be avoided, and meat should be a relatively minor part of the Pitta diet. Pittas are well suited to a vegetarian diet and thrive on fresh, unprocessed foods.

Every dosha trait has both positive and negative sides—positive when in balance, negative when not. The self-discipline of a Pitta can make losing a few pounds extremely easy, and it is this same quality that causes Pittas to thrive on exercise regimens that provide them with personal goals to fulfill. But if the Pitta dosha becomes imbalanced, the compulsion to self-destruct can be powerful; alcohol abuse, chronic overeating, and clinical eating disorders can develop if Pitta anger turns inward in the form of guilt. Yet the Pitta personality makes every effort to keep this inner turmoil from the view of others. Eating disorders such as anorexia are frequently seen in Pitta women who appear, at least on the surface, to be totally in control of their lives.

KAPHA

Characteristics of Kapha Type

- Solid, powerful build; great physical strength and endurance
- Steady energy; slow and graceful in action
- Tranquil, relaxed personality; slow to anger
- Cool, smooth, thick, pale, and often oily skin
- Slow to grasp new information, but good retentive memory
- Heavy, prolonged sleep
- Tendency toward obesity
- Slow digestion, mild hunger
- Affectionate, tolerant, forgiving
- Tendency to be possessive, complacent

It is very Kapha to
- Mull things over for a long time before making a decision
- Wake up slowly, lie in bed a long time, and need coffee upon arising

- Be happy with the status quo and preserve it by conciliat-ing others
- Respect other people's feelings (with which you feel gen-uine empathy)
- Seek emotional comfort from eating
- Have graceful movements, liquid eyes, and a gliding walk, even if overweight

Kapha people are of solid build, with great physical en-durance and strength. They move slowly and gracefully. Their skin is cool, smooth, and pale. Their digestion is slow, their hunger mild.

Kapha types tend to be tranquil, to have relaxed personali-ties, and to be slow to anger. Their sleep is heavy and prolonged, and they tend to become obese more often than the other body types. They're slow to grasp new information, but they have excellent retentive memory. Usually they're affectionate, toler-ant, and forgiving, but under stress they tend to become pos-sessive and complacent. The basic theme of the Kapha type is *relaxed*.

Kapha dosha, as the structural principle in the body, brings stability and steadiness to the physiology. It provides reserves of physical strength and stamina that have been built into the sturdy, heavy frames of typical Kapha types. Kaphas are con-sidered fortunate in Ayurveda because as a rule they enjoy sound health. Moreover, their personalities express a serene, happy, tranquil view of the world.

It is very Kapha to mull things over for a long time before making a decision, to wake up slowly, to lie in bed a long time, and perhaps to need coffee when they arise. Kapha types are happy with the status quo and preserve it by conciliating oth-ers. They respect the feelings of other people, with which they feel genuine empathy. They seek emotional comfort sometimes from eating, and this can be a problem. They have graceful movements, liquid eyes, and a gliding walk, even when they're overweight.

Ice cream, butter, milk, rich desserts, and other high-fat and very sweet foods should be avoided by those in whom the Kapha dosha is dominant. They should also avoid fried or oily foods. Light, warm foods should be favored instead. Most important of all, Kaphas should eat only when they're hungry, not just because it's lunchtime or because food is available. In fact, most Kapha types benefit from fasting one day a week, during which they avoid solid foods and take only fruit juices or skim milk. This results in greater overall energy and alertness.

Many Kapha types struggle with their weight all their lives, and this results in a sense of hopelessness and diminished self-esteem. But there's no reason to give up. Face the fact that a Kapha body simply does not conform to the media's ideal image of a hyperthin build, yet this in no way implies a lack of beauty or any other sort of inferiority. It's true that the Kapha's digestion and metabolism are inherently somewhat slow, and that Kaphas tend to lose weight more gradually than other people. But Ayurveda teaches that a balanced body is never overweight, and once Kapha types stabilize they will naturally return to their ideal weight.

YOUR BODY TYPE

At the end of this chapter you'll find a questionnaire that will help you determine your body type. But now that you have some idea of the three doshas, it should be clear that obesity is usually related to Kapha. Because this dosha governs the structure of the physiology, obesity will always involve imbalance of the Kapha dosha. But it is not uncommon for an imbalance in the Vata or Pitta doshas to precipitate the ultimate Kapha imbalance associated with obesity—an example of this would be nervous or compulsive eating. So regardless of which dosha is dominant in your physiology, you may be prone to obesity. Even a Vata type may end up being overweight.

Now you're ready to complete the Body-Type Questionnaire. Knowing your body type will allow you to get in touch with your inner intelligence and help you to respond more precisely to your internal signals. Let me be very clear about this, because I don't want you to think of the doshas as in any way defining the limits of your potential, the way lack of height might prevent you from being a professional basketball player. The doshas are a kind of fate, but only in the best possible sense. A correct understanding of your mind/body type gives you access to your genuine nature and to your healthy, beautiful, perfectly balanced self.

AYURVEDA BODY-TYPE QUESTIONNAIRE

The following quiz is divided into three sections. For the first 20 questions, which apply to Vata dosha, read each statement and mark, from 0 to 6, whether it applies to you.

    0 = Doesn't apply to me
    3 = Applies to me somewhat (or some of the time)
    6 = Applies to me mostly (or nearly all of the time)

At the end of the section, write down your total Vata score. For example, if you mark a 6 for the first question, a 3 for the second, and a 2 for the third, your total up to that point would be 6 + 3 + 2 = 11. Total the entire section in this way, and you arrive at your final Vata score. Proceed to the 20 questions for Pitta and those for Kapha.

When you are finished, you will have three separate scores. Comparing these will determine your body type.

For fairly objective physical traits, your choice will usually be obvious. For mental traits and behavior, which are more subjective, you should answer according to how you have felt and acted most of your life, or at least for the past few years.

SECTION 1: VATA

	Does not apply		Applies sometimes			Applies most	
1. I perform activity very quickly.	0	1	(2)	3	4	5	6
2. I am not good at memorizing things and then remembering them later.	0	1	2	3	(4)	5	6
3. I am enthusiastic and vivacious by nature.	0	1	2	3	(4)	5	6
4. I have a thin physique—I don't gain weight very easily.	(0)	1	2	3	4	5	6
5. I have always learned new things very quickly.	0	1	(2)	3	(4)	5	6
6. My characteristic gait while walking is light and quick.	0	1	(2)	3	4	5	6
7. I tend to have difficulty making decisions.	0	1	2	3	4	5	(6)
8. I tend to develop gas and become constipated easily.	0	1	2	3	4	5	(6)
9. I tend to have cold hands and feet.	0	1	(2)	3	4	5	6
10. I become anxious or worried frequently.	0	1	2	3	4	5	(6)
11. I don't tolerate cold weather as well as most people.	0	1	2	3	4	5	(6)
12. I speak quickly and my friends think that I'm talkative.	0	1	2	3	4	5	(6)
13. My moods change easily and I am somewhat emotional by nature.	0	1	2	(3)	4	5	6
14. I often have difficulty falling asleep or having a sound night's sleep.	0	(1)	2	3	4	5	6
15. My skin tends to be very dry, especially in winter.	0	1	2	3	4	5	(6)
16. My mind is very active, sometimes restless, but also very imaginative.	0	1	2	3	4	5	(6)
17. My movements are quick and active; my energy tends to come in bursts.	0	1	2	(3)	4	5	6

	Does not apply		Applies sometimes			Applies most
18. I am easily excitable.	0	1	2	3	4	5 6
19. I tend to be irregular in my eating and sleeping habits.	0	1	2	3	4	5 6
20. I learn quickly, but I also forget quickly.	0	1	2	3	4	5 6

VATA SCORE

SECTION 2: PITTA

	Does not apply		Applies sometimes			Applies most
1. I consider myself to be very efficient.	0	1	2	3	4	5 6
2. In my activities, I tend to be extremely precise and orderly.	0	1	2	3	4	5 6
3. I am strong-minded and have a somewhat forceful manner.	0	1	2	3	4	5 6
4. I feel uncomfortable or become easily fatigued in hot weather—more so than other people.	0	1	2	3	4	5 6
5. I tend to perspire easily.	0	1	2	3	4	5 6
6. Even though I might not always show it, I become irritable or angry quite easily.	0	1	2	3	4	5 6
7. If I skip a meal or a meal is delayed, I become uncomfortable.	0	1	2	3	4	5 6
8. One or more of the following characteristics describes my hair: • early graying or balding • thin, fine, straight • blond, red, or sandy-colored	0	1	2	3	4	5 6

	Does not apply		Applies sometimes				Applies most
9. I have a strong appetite; if I want to, I can eat quite a large quantity.	0	1	2	3	4	5	(6)
10. Many people consider me stubborn.	0	(1)	2	3	4	5	6
11. I am very regular in my bowel habits—it would be more common for me to have loose stools than to be constipated.	0	1	(2)	3	4	5	6
12. I become impatient very easily.	0	1	(2)	3	4	5	6
13. I tend to be a perfectionist about details.	0	(1)	2	3	4	5	6
14. I get angry quite easily, but then I quickly forget about it.	0	1	(2)	3	4	5	6
15. I am very fond of cold foods, such as ice cream, and also ice-cold drinks.	(0)	1	2	3	4	5	6
16. I am more likely to feel that a room is too hot than too cold.	0	1	2	3	(4)	5	6
17. I don't tolerate foods that are very hot and spicy.	0	(1)	2	3	4	5	6
18. I am not as tolerant of disagreement as I should be.	0	1	2	3	4	(5)	6
19. I enjoy challenges, and when I want something I am very determined in my efforts to get it.	0	1	2	3	(4)	5	6
20. I tend to be quite critical of others and also of myself.	0	1	2	3	(4)	5	6

PITTA SCORE

SECTION 3: KAPHA

	Does not apply		Applies sometimes			Applies most
1. My natural tendency is to do things in a slow and relaxed fashion.	0	1	2	3	4	5	**6**
2. I gain weight more easily than most people and lose it more slowly.	0	1	2	3	4	5	**6**
3. I have a placid and calm disposition—I'm not easily ruffled.	0	1	2	3	**4**	5	6
4. I can skip meals easily without any significant discomfort.	0	**1**	2	3	4	5	6
5. I have a tendency toward excess mucus or phlegm, chronic congestion, asthma, or sinus problems.	0	1	2	3	4	5	**6**
6. I must get at least eight hours of sleep in order to be comfortable the next day.	0	1	2	3	4	**5**	6
7. I sleep very deeply.	0	1	**2**	3	4	5	6
8. I am calm by nature and not easily angered.	0	1	2	3	**4**	5	6
9. I don't learn as quickly as some people, but I have excellent retention and a long memory.	0	1	2	3	**4**	5	6
10. I have a tendency toward becoming plump—I store extra fat easily.	0	1	2	3	4	5	**6**
11. Weather that is cool and damp bothers me.	0	1	**2**	3	4	5	6
12. My hair is thick, dark, and wavy.	**0**	1	2	3	4	5	6
13. I have smooth, soft skin with a somewhat pale complexion.	0	1	2	3	4	5	**6**
14. I have a large, solid body build.	0	1	2	3	4	5	**6**
15. The following words describe me well: serene, sweet-natured, affectionate, and forgiving.	0	1	2	3	**4**	5	6
16. I have slow digestion, which makes me feel heavy after eating.	0	1	2	3	4	**5**	6

	Does not apply			Applies sometimes			Applies most
17. I have very good stamina and physical endurance as well as a steady level of energy.	0	1	2	3	4	5	6
18. I generally walk with a slow, measured gait.	0	1	2	3	4	5	6
19. I have a tendency toward oversleeping and grogginess upon awakening, and am generally slow to get going in the morning.	0	1	2	3	4	5	6
20. I am a slow eater and am slow and methodical in my actions.	0	1	2	3	4	5	6

KAPHA SCORE

FINAL SCORE

VATA   **PITTA**   **KAPHA**

HOW TO DETERMINE YOUR BODY TYPE

Now that you have added up your scores, you can determine your body type. Although there are only three doshas, remember that Ayurveda combines them in ten ways to arrive at ten different body types.

• If one score is much higher than the others, you are probably a single-dosha type.

    Single-Dosha Types

    Vata

    Pitta

    Kapha

You are definitely a single-dosha type if one score is twice as high as another dosha score (for instance, Vata—90, Pitta—45, Kapha—35), but a smaller margin also applies. In single-dosha types, the characteristics of Vata, Pitta, or Kapha are very evident. Your next highest dosha will still show up in your natural tendencies, but it will be much less distinct.

• **If no single dosha dominates, you are a two-dosha type.**
 Two-Dosha Types
 Vata-Pitta or Pitta-Vata
 Pitta-Kapha or Kapha-Pitta
 Vata-Kapha or Kapha-Vata

If you are a two-dosha type, the traits of your two leading doshas will predominate. The higher one comes first in your body type, but both count.

Most people are two-dosha types. A two-dosha type might have a score like this: Vata—80, Pitta—90, Kapha—20. If this was your score, you would consider yourself to be a Pitta-Vata type.

• **If your three scores are nearly equal, you may be a three-dosha type.**
 Three-Dosha
 Vata-Pitta-Kapha

However, this type is considered to be the rarest of all. Check your answers again, or have a friend go over your responses with you. Also, you can read over the descriptions of Vata, Pitta, and Kapha included in this chapter to see if one or two doshas are more prominent in your makeup.

3

MASTERING THE KEY

TO WEIGHT LOSS

For millions of years, the struggle to get enough food was the first priority of the human species. Survival depended on it, and societies were organized around it. During periods when food was abundant, it was natural and prudent for people to eat as much as possible, since there was sure to be a period of scarcity in the near future. In accord with this cycle of feast and famine, the human body evolved a process of saving food that was not immediately metabolized as energy: it was stored in the form of fat. Obviously, this was a very successful adaptive mechanism of the human physiology. Stored fat meant that the species could endure extended periods of scarcity without starving to death.

Today, at least in some parts of the world, the cycle of feast and famine has ended. In more fortunate countries we can eat whenever we want, as much as we want, for as long as we want. But the chemistry of the body has not yet adapted to this change. The body is still endlessly preparing for a period of scarcity that it thinks may be just around the corner. It continues to store as fat whatever is not quickly used as energy.

This is not a disease. This is normal and natural. Your weight right now is the natural outcome of what you eat combined with the energy requirements of your lifestyle and the persistent effects of millions of years of human evolution.

Even if you drastically altered both your eating habits and your level of daily exercise, you might still be overweight by the standards of contemporary fashion. There are two reasons for this. First, the standards of fashion are greatly out of line with the structure of most people. Second, your body can't tell the difference between food deprivation that occurs in order to fit into smaller-size blue jeans and deprivation caused by famine or other catastrophe. In either case, the body goes into a "starvation mode" of lowered metabolism, in which fat is burned more slowly. Remember: This is an extremely powerful mechanism that has evolved over the entire span of human history. It's very difficult to change.

All of this means that being overweight or being at your natural weight is a more subjective matter than you may have recognized. If you've been eating a quart of chocolate ice cream every day, you may have found a way to rationalize this, but you probably know that this is not what nature intended, for an imbalance occurs. If you want to correct that imbalance and get back into synchronization with the perfection of your original design, you can certainly do so. But if you attempt to go beyond the perfection of your design *in the other direction*, by trying to duplicate the physique of someone fundamentally different from you, you will be battling against biological forces that are extremely difficult to master, especially over extended periods of time.

Therefore, effective weight control involves at least two important components: recognizing and eliminating behaviors resulting from imbalances, and acknowledging, accepting, and enjoying what *is* your true nature. The purpose of this chapter is to help you do both these things.

BALANCING YOUR SYSTEM

Overweight represents a general imbalance in the physiology, which is another way of saying that a weight problem is not just a problem of weight. If we focus merely on the loss of weight and measure progress only in terms of pounds and inches, success will always be limited because we haven't dealt with the underlying imbalance.

Simply losing weight will never create a state of perfect balance for the physiology, but creating perfect balance will always result in a spontaneous, completely positive outcome: Your weight will go to the level that is normal and natural for you. But if you start following external cues again, it can result only in a state of imbalance all over again.

Very often, when we decide to lose weight, what we really want is to be more beautiful, more attractive, more lively, or more energetic. Yet when people perceive these qualities in one another, they aren't really perceived in actual weight. Ayurveda says that outer beauty depends on inner beauty. And inner beauty is a spontaneous and effortless result of perfect balance of mind and body.

Creating this balance simply means reconnecting our physiology with the intelligence of nature already within us. It means removing any obstacles to the full expression of that intelligence. To use Ayurvedic terminology, it means balancing the three doshas so that the flow of intelligence is perfect throughout the physiology.

Michelangelo's genius as a sculptor lay in his ability to see a finished statue inside a rough block of marble. His challenge was not to make a sculpture but to release the one that was already there, imprisoned in the stone. Essentially, this is what you do when you bring yourself back into balance. Instead of creating a "new" you, a thinner you, you are simply *releasing* a hidden you. The process is one of personal discovery. The hidden you that wants to emerge is already in perfect balance. Finding it is not a rote affair, and every person achieves balance in his or her own way. Like hunger and thirst, the instinct for balance is built into your very physiology. Once you begin to follow that instinct for balance, the perfection of your true nature will shine through.

Of course, all this is really a matter of self-acceptance. Self-acceptance is the precondition for genuine physical beauty as well as emotional happiness and spiritual fulfillment. To put it another way, *lack* of self-acceptance is the basis for a large portion of human misery and self-destructive behavior. This is what leads people to attempt to camouflage their problems, whether by using expensive cosmetics or eating too many candy bars. Yet all of us know individuals who, even though they may not meet conventional standards of physical attractiveness, shine with the special radiance that is the expression of self-acceptance. As you contemplate making changes in your life, be sure that they're based on a solid foundation of positive feelings about yourself, and not on an attempt to live up to someone else's notion of what you should be. Your understanding of that distinction can be the critical difference between success and disappointment when you implement a weight control program. Remember: In Ayurveda, nothing is simply a mechanical or a technical procedure. Your motives and your feelings are as important as whatever you do or don't do.

Imbalanced Vata

- Dry or rough skin
- Insomnia
- Constipation

- Common fatigue
- Tension headaches
- Intolerance of cold
- Degenerative arthritis
- Underweight
- Anxiety, worry

Imbalanced Pitta

- Rashes, inflammatory skin diseases
- Peptic ulcer, heartburn
- Visual problems
- Excessive body heat
- Premature graying or baldness
- Hostility, irritability

Imbalanced Kapha

- Overweight/obesity
- Slow digestion
- Allergies, sinus congestion, runny nose
- Dullness, depression
- Laziness, lethargy
- Asthma
- Joint problems

HOMEOSTASIS

Every function in your body has a natural level it wants to return to, just as a thermostat has its set point. The medical term for this is *homeostasis*. You can raise your body's temperature by running half a mile or sitting in a sauna, for example, but after you stop, your temperature will return to 98.6 degrees F. This is home base for your body's thermostat, and if you depart from it too far or too long, you will experience unpleasant repercussions.

One of the reasons for the complexity of humans is that hundreds of thermostats have been installed inside us, each obeying its own set of natural laws. The body has many balance points, not just one, and the coordination among them is quite miraculous. You may think of the bloodstream as a random swirl of biochemicals, considering the bewildering number of hormones, nutrients, and diverse messenger molecules that flow through it. But in fact the bloodstream is so exactly balanced that all these molecules go where they're needed with exquisitely precise timing and in exact measure.

Similarly, the brain is capable of keeping track of all our biological functions without confusion. One tiny portion of gray matter in the forebrain, called the *hypothalamus*, weighing roughly one-sixth of an ounce, is responsible for balancing an amazing number of diverse operations, including fat and carbohydrate metabolism, sleeping and waking, appetite, thirst, digestive secretions, levels of fluids, growth, and body temperature. In short, the hypothalamus controls everything that goes on automatically in the body, including all the factors that determine your weight.

Physiological balance is a function of intelligence. We are much more than a collection of thermostats, because a thermostat cannot set itself, and we can. The original setting you were born with is your *prakriti*, your body type. At birth the ideal balance point for the three doshas is set for the person's lifetime.

Just as the automatic functions of the body obey the hypothalamus, all of the hundreds of thermostats in the body obey the master setting of the doshas. But there's a crucial difference: you can influence and communicate with your doshas, but you cannot do so with your hypothalamus. Vata levels, predictably, go up in the presence of any aggravating influence such as cold weather, dry moving air, fear, spicy food, and staying up too late at night; all these factors aggravate Vata. These behaviors say "more Vata" to the body. In the same way, Pitta and Kapha have their own catalysts.

Imbalances that accumulate over time move us away from our prakriti, or our own true destiny. These imbalances are called *vikriti* in Ayurveda, a Sanskrit word that means "deviating from nature." Thus the two terms, prakriti and vikriti, are opposites, one referring to what is natural for a person, the other to what is not. The wrong food, poor sleeping habits, negative emotions, and physical and/or mental strain make life a bit less natural and eventually result in physical symptoms, diseases, and problems such as overweight. There's an emotional side to this as well. Self-destructive habits change positive emotional responses to negative ones. In short, vikriti makes us more sensitive to stresses of all kinds.

But vikriti, or imbalance, is really an illusion built on harmful assumptions. One of the most perilous of these assumptions, something we've come to take for granted, is the concept of ego. By this I mean the belief that you are an individual entity, fundamentally separate from the universe. This is a conditioned belief, a product of your culture—a mere point of view, not a biological absolute. Your body has no definite beginning in time and space, and it is not moving toward some predetermined end. Your physiology is constantly remaking itself every second, and will continue to do so as long as it exists. Exactly *how* it continues to do so can be directly influenced by signals your brain sends in regard to everything you do: your job, your relationships, and certainly what you eat. If you continue to replay the same negative thoughts and feelings that have burdened you for many years, you will continue to have the same physiology. Fortunately, however, you can change all that. Underneath those negative habits is something very different and inherently beautiful; below the surface of your life is that original, ideal setting, the unique combination of Vata, Pitta, and Kapha doshas that is the real you. If that combination can be recovered, overweight and any other problems will spontaneously disappear. This is the beauty of Ayurveda, which makes people healthy by returning them to their true, natural selves.

THE IMPORTANCE OF A DAILY ROUTINE

As I've mentioned, the most common factor associated with obesity is an imbalance of Kapha. This is true regardless of your primary body type. Although this book provides methods for balancing all three doshas, I'll give special attention to correcting imbalance in the Kapha dosha. These techniques will help you not only in losing weight but in creating more energy, vitality, and bliss.

I will devote the rest of this chapter to the importance of a stabilized daily routine. Every day the sun rises and sets, and countless different things happen in between. Nature is so beautifully arranged that no matter how different these things are, they seem to fit into one rhythm. But actually there are rhythms nestled inside one another, like wheels within wheels.

Modern medicine has disclosed many of the obvious cycles in our bodies: the heart beating every three quarters of a second, the lungs swelling to inhale air ten to fourteen times a minute; however, many of the body's changes remain quite mysterious. Why does our body typically weigh the most at seven in the evening? Why are our hands hottest at two in the morning? Research has unearthed these facts, but as yet we have no explanations. Ayurveda's rationale is that every day we pass through various master cycles. We feel the influence of these cycles in terms of Kapha, Pitta and Vata. These three cycles take place from sunrise to sunset, and then they repeat themselves again from sunset to sunrise. The approximate times for these cycles are represented in the following diagram:

MASTER CYCLES OF VATA, PITTA, AND KAPHA

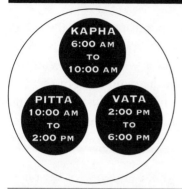

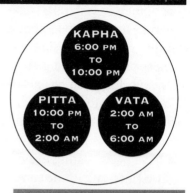

FIRST CYCLE

Kapha predominates from
　　6:00 A.M. to 10:00 A.M.
Pitta predominates from
　　10:00 A.M. to 2:00 P.M.
Vata predominates from
　　2:00 P.M. to 6:00 P.M.

SECOND CYCLE

Kapha predominates from
　　6:00 P.M. to 10:00 P.M.
Pitta predominates from
　　10:00 P.M. to 2:00 A.M.
Vata predominates from
　　2:00 A.M. to 6:00 A.M.

One of the most basic aspects of living in tune with nature is to respect these master cycles that support our physical existence. We are meant to ride nature's waves, not to fight against them. In fact, our bodies are already riding them, or at least doing the best they can in the face of our contrary habits.

In the late evening, as the sun is setting, it seems as if all of nature is settling down. Everyone feels comfortable sitting back and relaxing after a day's work. The birds are going to sleep, and there is a sense of heaviness in the air. By the end of the Kapha cycle at 10:00 P.M., some people may notice that they feel ready for sleep.

Likewise, if we examine the main Pitta period of the day— from 10:00 A.M. to 2:00 P.M.—we find it's the time when we feel like being physically active and when appetite is greatest. This is because the Pitta dosha is responsible for metabolizing food, for distributing energy, and for more efficient physical functioning in general.

Pitta's function in the body corresponds to that of the sun in nature. So when the sun is at its peak around noon, the body is most prepared to digest food. This is why, in most cultures in the world, lunch has always been the main meal of the day. It is actually only since nations have become industrialized, and people have begun to build their basic biological routines around their work rather than the other way around, that people have begun eating heavy dinners.

You can think of the sun as a kind of a support for the physical function of digestion. When the sun is high in the sky, there is more support for the body's digestive processes. Likewise, when the sun is rising in the morning and setting in the evening, digestive capacity is weaker because there is less support from the environment for the Pitta in the body. *So an extremely important Ayurvedic recommendation is to take your heaviest meal at lunchtime. Moreover, you should take that meal at approximately the same time each day, in the middle of the Pitta period.*

By taking your lunch at about noon or 12:30 P.M., you can digest even a large quantity of food and assimilate it properly. This will generate maximum energy and will therefore help avoid the need to have a large dinner, which is more difficult to digest, digestion being less keen in the evening. This one very simple change will actually make a profound difference in your metabolism. Because digestion is stronger at midday, it is more efficient in converting food into energy instead of into fat. Eating should produce energy, vitality, and bliss, rather than fat and impurities that are stored in the physiology and are difficult to get rid of.

If you work during the day, it may be difficult or inconvenient to make lunch your largest meal. But ensuring a proper lunch each day can greatly enhance your progress toward reawakening the physiological intelligence within you. More-over, at lunch each day you should focus not on calories, not on quantity, but on the *quality* of the food. It should be wholesome, nutritious, delicious, and freshly cooked. And re-member to stop eating when you reach level 6 on your Satisfaction Meter.

EATING LUNCH AT THE SAME TIME EVERY DAY

In chapter 1, I asked you to eat only when you felt hungry. That instruction was to be followed for the first two weeks of your Ayurvedic weight control program; its purpose was to assist your body in eliminating impurities and to make you aware of your hunger and eating patterns. After fourteen days I would like you to switch to a pattern of taking lunch at the same time every day and making this your heaviest meal. If you follow the instructions in this book, you'll find that soon you will auto-matically feel hungry at about the same time each day, which, as I said, should be at noon or half an hour later. Make this mealtime part of your regular, permanent routine.

What about other meals? For most people following this program, the best routine will be to take little or no breakfast. Unlike Western medicine, Ayurveda considers breakfast to be an optional meal, not a necessary one. However, the most im-portant overall principle is to do nothing that produces dis-comfort in your physiology. Those who have strong appetites, especially those who have predominantly Pitta constitutions, may require a light breakfast of milk and cereal or tea and toast in order to be comfortable until lunchtime. If you are in the habit of eating a heavy breakfast, however, switch to a lighter one, which should give you a greater appetite at lunchtime. You'll find you'll feel more alert, energetic, and comfortable all day as a result.

In general, by taking a well-balanced, solid lunch, you won't be as hungry later. Therefore dinner should be lighter, but it should not be skipped. By "light" I'm referring to two things: the food should not be inherently substantial, such as meat or a heavy pasta-based casserole, and the quantity consumed should be less than at lunch. Some examples of dinners that you may find very satisfying are hot soup and bread, hot cereals, vegetables and grains, light casseroles, and so on. Meats, especially red meats, are better taken at lunch than at dinner.

In chapter 1, you were advised to eat only when you reached level 0 to 1. You were asked to maintain this routine for two weeks, using the **Daily Record of Hunger Levels** table to record your progress. Once the two weeks are over, start this routine:

BREAKFAST

Skip breakfast or eat a light breakfast such as milk and cereal or juice and toast.

LUNCH

Make lunch the heaviest meal of the day. Eat at about the same time each day, around noon or 12:30 P.M. Do not focus on the calories or quantity of food, but on the quality. It should be freshly cooked, wholesome, nutritious, and delicious.

DINNER

Eat dinner daily, but eat smaller amounts and lighter foods than at lunch. A typical dinner could be hot soup and bread, hot cereals, vegetables and grains, or light casseroles. Avoid meats at night.

CREATING A SUCCESSFUL DAILY ROUTINE

This point about eating the heaviest meal at lunchtime is the most important aspect of the Ayurvedic daily routine when it comes to dealing with weight loss. However, there are other elements of the Ayurvedic routine that are worth emphasizing.

One point has to do with bedtime. A tired body is one that is not alert to its inner needs. Remember that a Kapha period occurs from about 6:00 to 10:00 P.M., and that some of the qualities of the Kapha dosha are heaviness, slowness, and dullness. This means that at this time there is support from nature to settle down and go to sleep.

Ten o'clock in the evening is an important junction between the influence of Kapha and that of Pitta in the environment. While Kapha is heavy, slow, and dull, Pitta is light, sharp, and hot, with heat representing activity. As a result of this switch to Pitta-dominant time, you may have noticed that if you stay up until 10:30 P.M. or later, you get a second wind that lets you easily stay up until 12:30 or even 2:00 A.M., still feeling somewhat fresh.

But when you do this, either you must set an alarm in order to get up on time in the morning, which can cause you to feel tired, or else you'll oversleep. If you do oversleep, until 8:00 or 9:00 A.M. or even later, you will rise during the next Kapha period, which occurs between 6:00 and 10:00 A.M.

Remember the qualities of Kapha? Heavy, slow, and dull. That is exactly how you'll feel if you arise at that time. In addition, some of this excess Kapha influence, which would not have been in effect if you had arisen at the proper time, will stay with you all day and make your job of losing weight even more difficult. In my practice, I've noticed that people who arise late in the morning tend to feel less energetic and have a higher incidence of depression.

If you go to bed early—by about 10:00 P.M.—you'll naturally

arise earlier in the morning. The closer you can come to arising before the end of the Vata period (6:00 A.M.), the better off you'll be. If you arise before the influence of Vata has completely left the environment, you'll feel light, energetic, and quick. What's more, you'll feel this way all day as a result of this simple switch in your routine.

One other very valuable addition to your daily routine involves special types of massage. The first is called *garshan*, which is a dry massage. Ayurveda recommends it specifically for weight loss because it stimulates circulation and helps the body to eliminate impurities. Experience has shown that this massage also helps to eliminate cellulite. The second massage, called *abhyanga*, uses sesame oil. Ayurveda recommends this sesame-oil massage as part of the daily routine for everyone, because it rejuvenates and revitalizes the physiology. It produces a youthful influence for the skin and helps to balance all three doshas.

As you lose weight, these special massages will help to keep your skin toned and firm and to prevent wrinkles and sagging skin. Try to incorporate both massages into your daily routine before your morning bath. They take only a few minutes each, and you'll feel fresher and more vital all day. If you don't have time to do them every day, try for at least three times a week. Or, if you prefer, do the dry massage only.

How to Do Garshan Massage

Garshan is an Ayurvedic dry massage for stimulating blood flow and circulation through all the tissues of your body. This simple purification procedure washes away impurities and helps facilitate weight loss. It helps with digestion, metabolism, and the reduction of cellulite.

Garshan takes only three to four minutes. The best time to do it is in the morning before your bath. Garshan precedes the oil massage. Ideally, garshan is performed with a pair of raw silk gloves. Otherwise, use a loofa as an alternative. Loofas are available at health food stores.

1. Put on your silk gloves.
2. Throughout the massage, use fairly vigorous strokes. Use long strokes back and forth over the long bones of your body. Use circular strokes over your joints. You may find that you can gradually increase the number of strokes over the long bones from ten or twenty up to a maximum of forty.
3. Start by massaging your head, then move down your neck and shoulder area. Use circular movements over your shoulder joints, long strokes over your upper arms, circular movements over your elbows, long strokes over your forearms, circular movements over your wrists, long strokes over your hands, and circular movements over your joints.
4. Move to the chest area next. Avoid massaging directly over your heart and breasts. On your upper chest, use long, horizontal strokes, moving back and forth.
5. On your abdomen, stroke back and forth twice horizontally, then twice diagonally. You'll want to spend a little more time on the areas where there is an accumulation of fat, such as the abdomen, thighs, buttocks, and arms.
6. Stand up at this point. Go over your hip area vigorously. Then use long strokes over your thighs, circular strokes over your knees, long strokes over your calves, circular strokes over your ankles, and long strokes over your feet.

How to Do Ayurvedic Oil Massage

Ayurvedic oil massage (abhyanga) helps strengthen and balance your whole body, improves circulation and vitality, and rejuvenates your skin.

1. Start with cold-pressed sesame oil, available from your health food store. Ideally, the oil should be "cured" before using. (Instructions for curing are given on page 55) The oil should be warmed each day before you use it. One easy way to do this is to keep the oil in a small plastic bottle with a flip-top lid. Warm the oil by placing the bottle in a sink or container filled with hot water for a few minutes.

2. Use the open part of your hand (rather than your fingertips) to massage your entire body. In general, use circular motions over rounded areas (joints, head) and straight strokes over straight areas (neck, long bones). Apply moderate pressure over most of your body and light pressure over your abdomen and heart.

3. Start with your head. Pour a small amount of oil on your hands and vigorously massage it into your scalp. With the flat part of your hands, use circular strokes to cover your whole head. Spend more time massaging your head than other parts of your body.

4. Next, massage your face and outer ears, remembering to apply a small amount of oil as you move from one part of your body to the next. Massage this area more gently.

5. Massage the front and back of your neck and the upper part of your spine. At this point you may want to cover the rest of your body with a thin layer of oil to give maximum time for the oil to soak in.

6. Vigorously massage your arms, using a circular motion on your shoulders and elbows and long, back-and-forth strokes on your upper arms and forearms.

7. Now massage your chest and stomach. Use a very gentle, circular motion over your heart and abdomen. You can start in the lower right part of your abdomen and move clockwise, ending up at the lower left part. This gently massages your intestines.

8. Massage your back and spine. You may have trouble reaching your entire back.

9. Massage your legs vigorously, using circular motions over your hips, knees, and ankles. Use long, straight strokes over your thighs and calves.

10. Finally, massage the bottoms of your feet. As with your head, this important area of your body deserves more time. Use the palm of your hand to massage your soles vigorously.

11. Follow your oil massage with a warm bath or shower, using a mild soap.

How to Prepare Sesame Oil for Ayurvedic Oil Massage

Ayurveda recommends using unprocessed, cold-pressed sesame oil, which is available at health food stores. Before using the sesame oil, it's best to cure the oil by following these simple steps. Curing increases the oil's ability to penetrate the skin.

1. Heat the oil to about the boiling temperature of water (212° F). To know when the oil is hot enough, simply add a single drop of water to the oil before you heat it. When the water crackles or boils on top of the oil, you can remove the oil from the heat. Or just observe the oil as it heats. When it begins to move and circulate in the pan, remove it from the burner.

2. If you like, you can cure up to one quart of oil at a time. This should be enough for at least two weeks.

3. Because all oils are flammable, be sure to observe proper safety precautions. Use **low** rather than high heat, never leave the room while the oil is heating, and remove the oil promptly once the proper temperature is reached. Be sure to store the oil in a safe place when cooling, out of the reach of children.

4

Using the Power of Your Digestion to Lose Weight

In learning to control your weight you must keep in mind that hunger—meaning proper appetite—is your friend, not your enemy. By taking advantage of this fact, you can digest your food in a way that automatically produces lean tissue instead of excess fat.

In chapter 1 we saw that our bodies are not frozen statues, fixed in space and time, and that at every moment we are regenerating the intelligence of the physiology, actually rebuilding every cell and sinew every second of every day. But how does this actually take place on a material level? Specifically, it is accomplished through digestion.

It is through the foods we eat that we extract intelligence from the environment, and we metabolize that intelligence so that it can be used by our bodies. Eating is the most direct expression of our intimate connection with the environment. Each time we eat we process food through a wonderfully sophisticated and intricate series of biochemical events that transform that material from the environment into our physical being.

We'll deal with which foods are best to eat in a later chapter. For the present we're more concerned with what happens before and after we eat than we are with the food itself. We want to understand the mechanics of appetite and digestion.

In my medical practice I've learned that if I ask an overweight patient about his or her appetite, I nearly always get the same response. First the patient gives a little chuckle, then he or she says, "My appetite is much too good!" This response reveals the almost universal belief of overweight people that appetite and hunger are their enemies. Through the years, through innumerable diets and fads, these people have struggled against their bodies' natural cravings. They have fought these cravings with an arsenal of weapons including pills, diet books and programs, fiber supplements, and anything else they could think of. I believe all such efforts are thoroughly misguided. When we fight our appetite, we are fighting nature. It is not only a useless fight but a hopeless one.

Where does hunger come from? Ayurveda explains that hunger comes from the digestive fires known as *agnis*. Agni literally means "fire." Ayurveda describes the process of digestion in terms of heat, as if the food is actually being burned before it is further processed. When you compare the Ayurvedic description to what is known in modern biochemistry and physiology, the two concepts are quite consistent. When you're hungry, then the fires, the agni, are burning hotter. This means they are best prepared to digest and assimilate food. It is our agni, or our digestive capacity, that allows us properly to assimilate the foods we eat and convert them into energy rather than into fat and toxins.

According to Ayurveda, imperfections in digestion are always present in people who have chronic weight problems. Ayurveda describes a product of improper digestion *ama*. Ama is both an abstract principle and a material element. Materially, it is a white, sticky substance that clogs all the normal channels of flow in the physiology. These channels are not only for the passage of blood and lymph but for normal energy. Because it blocks the channels of circulation in the physiology, ama is an extremely common precursor of a wide variety of diseases, and it causes the symptoms so common to overweight people: lethargy, dullness, erratic eating habits, compulsive eating, distortion of hunger sensations, and obesity itself.

All this is not really very far from the thinking of contemporary Western medicine, in which the notion of debris building up in the cells has long been accepted. This cellular debris is thought to interfere with the correct functioning of DNA and is thus implicated in the etiology of cancer and the aging process. But beyond acknowledging its destructive effects, Western medicine is still rather vague about the characteristics of this waste matter in the cells, while Ayurveda is quite specific about ama.

You can literally see ama. How many times have you noticed a white coating on your tongue, especially just after you've awakened? This is ama, and if it is present on your tongue, it is present throughout your physiology.

It is highly impractical to treat any imbalance of the physiology when ama is present—and it is extremely difficult, perhaps impossible, to lose weight. This is why so many people who have limited their diets to the point of virtual starvation still have failed to accomplish their goals. Therefore it's essential to take practical steps to eliminate ama in order to lose weight and keep it off permanently. Ama is, quite simply, a key in the pathogenesis of obesity. After all, one of the principle qualities of ama is *heaviness*.

Foods that are of salty, sour, or sweet taste are especially implicated in accumulation of ama. Dietary changes, herbal therapies, and fasting are especially beneficial in eliminating it.

But ama has a positive counterpart that can also be present throughout the body. By eating properly and following the correct routines, this different and opposite product of digestion, called *ojas*, can be formed. Ayurveda describes ojas as the bio-chemical equivalent of bliss. Think about that for a moment. By creating ojas within your physiology, you are literally storing up the physical manifestation of joy and total well-being. What could be more important? What could be of greater benefit to your overall health?

When you take steps to eliminate ama, more ojas is automatically produced. Likewise, by taking steps to enhance ojas, you will create less ama. So it is useful to know the symptoms of both these important substances. After eating a particular meal or following particular routines, if you feel the symptoms relating to ama, then you know that something was wrong in the food or the routine. But if you feel the symptoms of ojas following a particular routine, you know that your physiology is being nourished and balanced by that action. Let's itemize the symptoms of each:

> **Evidence of ama:** weakness, heaviness, lethargy, poor immunity, irregular elimination, fatigue, fluctuations in appetite, energy level, and mood. There is commonly a white coating on the tongue, especially in the morning on arising.
>
> **Evidence of ojas:** lightness of body, excellent energy, strong appetite and digestion, perfect immunity, regular elimination, physical strength and stamina, and a general sense of bliss. Both physically and mentally, there is an experience of vitality and intense well-being.

Before we discuss nutrition and the foods that result in ojas and ama, I want to introduce some extremely important techniques to eliminate ama from the system by strengthening the digestion and maintaining that strength throughout life. I call these Body Intelligence Techniques. They're simple ways to enliven the body's own inner intelligence so that food can be digested into energy, intelligence, and bliss. Some of the techniques will require you to change some of your present habits, but the benefits of doing so will be immediate and obvious.

BODY INTELLIGENCE TIPS

Eat in a settled and quiet atmosphere. The conditions under which food is consumed are as important as the food itself. Don't divide your attention by working, reading, listening to the radio, or watching television during meals. When you eat, your attention should be on the food, so that you can savor all the delightful flavors and truly enjoy your food. Overweight people tend to wolf down their meals without respect or attention. They often rely on fast food restaurants, where the pace and hectic atmosphere is the opposite of a healthy environment for eating.

Always sit down to eat. Even if you're going to have a snack, consisting perhaps of a few grapes or raisins, take the time to sit down at the table. Pay attention to what you're doing, and don't rush. This will help to prepare your digestion and to enforce your awareness of the food and your hunger level.

Don't eat when you're upset. If you're upset, disturbed, or angry at mealtime, this will definitely disturb the digestion and produce ama. It is best to postpone the meal a few minutes until you feel more settled.

Eat only up to the point of comfort. Remember level 6 on your Satisfaction Meter. Ayurveda says we should eat up to about three-fourths of our capacity. Eating beyond this level is like trying to kindle a fire and then smothering it with too much fuel just as the fire is getting started. A smothered digestive fire produces ama.

Avoid ice-cold foods and drinks. Cold foods and drinks tend to freeze the digestive fires, thus allowing the food to be converted into ama. This is especially true of ice-cold foods and drinks. In addition, because both Vata and Kapha are cold by nature, these two doshas will be disturbed by cold foods and drinks. In the treatment of obesity, the Vata and Kapha doshas are the ones most in need of being brought into balance. Many people find that it takes time to break the habit of choosing ice-cold drinks. But within a few weeks you'll find you no longer miss those cold drinks, and your body will feel much better without them.

Don't talk while chewing. When chewing and swallowing, your senses should be focused inward, enjoying the taste, sight, and aroma of food. In any case, conversations at the dinner table should be light and settled in nature, not emotional or disruptive.

Eat at a moderate pace. To help regulate your speed, don't place the next bite of food on your fork or spoon until the preceding bite has been chewed and swallowed.

Don't eat until the preceding meal has been fully digested. Digestion usually takes three to six hours to complete. Continuing to snack while you are still digesting the preceding meal will produce ama. If you feel that you must have a snack, make it something light, like a piece of fruit or a small glass of fruit juice.

Favor meals with freshly cooked foods. Most people think that eating more raw foods will help them lose weight. While a certain quantity of raw foods in the diet is fine, cooked foods generally are easier to digest and less likely to produce ama than raw foods are. Most of your meals should be cooked, soothing, balanced, and delicious. Also, the food should be freshly cooked; leftovers often have a heavier quality, which makes them more difficult to digest and more likely to produce ama.

Sit quietly for a few minutes after your meal. This allows digestion to begin effortlessly. It also shows respect for the act of eating and for the metabolic processes that are set in motion by it. Even if your work requires you to "eat and run," the brief period you devote to relaxation immediately after eating will be time well spent. Those few moments express a critical difference in your approach to eating and to your health in general.

Finally, devote one or two meals each week to what I call Eating Awareness Meditation. This is a technique for using the power of intention to improve digestion and metabolism. It should be done when you are eating alone. The technique involves eating very slowly and deliberately, while consciously *intending* every movement.

Begin by looking at the food with an awareness of the intention to look at it. Become aware of the food's aroma by having the intention of being aware of it. When you taste each bite, intend to taste it. We have become used to eating quickly and automatically, as if we were dialing a telephone or paying a utility bill. Ayurveda states: "A person eating in ignorance can make poison of any food." But by taking one or two meals a week with awareness and intention, you can gradually improve your whole attitude toward nourishing your body. Eating Awareness Meditation is absolutely essential to practice and to master.

NOTE: Some of the Body Intelligence Techniques may require some effort at the outset. This is often the case when revising lifelong habits that are not beneficial to health, such as watching television or reading while eating. These habits make us less aware of our eating, produce ama in our physiology, and make it difficult for us to lose weight.

At the end of this chapter you'll find a checklist to help you incorporate the Body Intelligence Techniques into your daily routine. If some of them are difficult to undertake immediately, begin with the ones that are simplest; then add another technique each week until you've got them all.

By making these techniques part of your daily routine, you will be bringing the act of eating into your conscious awareness. By doing so, you will also bring life-centered, present-moment focus into your daily experience. This increases your enjoyment not only of food but of everything you do.

In this chapter you've learned some powerful ways to strengthen digestion so that food is converted into the vital tissues of the physiology rather than into wasteful fat. Next, you'll learn more specifics about diet and which foods will actually help to eliminate fat from your system.

Start using your **Checklist** every time you eat, whether it is a full meal or a snack. This will help you monitor your progress in applying the techniques. If some of them seem too difficult, try the easy one s first. Then add a new technique every week until you have incorporated them all.

BODY INTELLIGENCE TECHNIQUES CHECKLIST

Use this checklist every time you eat. For the **first** meal of the day, use the circles numbered with a 1 to check off the techniques you used. If you did not use a Body Intelligence Technique, leave the space blank. There are enough spaces to record four meals or snacks a day.

	Monday	Tuesday	Wednesday	Thursday	Friday	Saurday	Sunday
Ate in a settled and quiet atmosphere	1○ 2○ 3○ 4○	1○ 2○ 3○ 4○	1○ 2○ 3○ 4○	1○ 2○ 3○ 4○	1○ 2○ 3○ 4○	1○ 2○ 3○ 4○	1○ 2○ 3○ 4○
Sat down at a table to eat	1○ 2○ 3○ 4○	1○ 2○ 3○ 4○	1○ 2○ 3○ 4○	1○ 2○ 3○ 4○	1○ 2○ 3○ 4○	1○ 2○ 3○ 4○	1○ 2○ 3○ 4○
Didn't eat when upset	1○ 2○ 3○ 4○	1○ 2○ 3○ 4○	1○ 2○ 3○ 4○	1○ 2○ 3○ 4○	1○ 2○ 3○ 4○	1○ 2○ 3○ 4○	1○ 2○ 3○ 4○
Stopped eating at level 6	1○ 2○ 3○ 4○	1○ 2○ 3○ 4○	1○ 2○ 3○ 4○	1○ 2○ 3○ 4○	1○ 2○ 3○ 4○	1○ 2○ 3○ 4○	1○ 2○ 3○ 4○

Avoided cold food and drinks	1○ 2○ 3○ 4○	1○ 2○ 3○ 4○	1○ 2○ 3○ 4○	1○ 2○ 3○ 4○	1○ 2○ 3○ 4○	1○ 2○ 3○ 4○	1○ 2○ 3○ 4○
Didn't talk while chewing	1○ 2○ 3○ 4○	1○ 2○ 3○ 4○	1○ 2○ 3○ 4○	1○ 2○ 3○ 4○	1○ 2○ 3○ 4○	1○ 2○ 3○ 4○	1○ 2○ 3○ 4○
Ate at a moderate pace	1○ 2○ 3○ 4○	1○ 2○ 3○ 4○	1○ 2○ 3○ 4○	1○ 2○ 3○ 4○	1○ 2○ 3○ 4○	1○ 2○ 3○ 4○	1○ 2○ 3○ 4○
Ate after the preceding meal had been completely digested	1○ 2○ 3○ 4○	1○ 2○ 3○ 4○	1○ 2○ 3○ 4○	1○ 2○ 3○ 4○	1○ 2○ 3○ 4○	1○ 2○ 3○ 4○	1○ 2○ 3○ 4○
Ate a freshly cooked and balanced meal	1○ 2○ 3○ 4○	1○ 2○ 3○ 4○	1○ 2○ 3○ 4○	1○ 2○ 3○ 4○	1○ 2○ 3○ 4○	1○ 2○ 3○ 4○	1○ 2○ 3○ 4○
Sat quietly for a few minutes after eating	1○ 2○ 3○ 4○	1○ 2○ 3○ 4○	1○ 2○ 3○ 4○	1○ 2○ 3○ 4○	1○ 2○ 3○ 4○	1○ 2○ 3○ 4○	1○ 2○ 3○ 4○

5

EATING RIGHT

WITHOUT DIETING

Strict dieting, in the sense of counting calories and severely restricting the intake of food, can actually cause you to gain weight rather than lose it, particularly over long periods of time. Only about 20 percent of people who lose weight through dieting are able to keep it off for at least a year. And, as previously mentioned, the effect on health of losing and regaining pounds is worse than being overweight in the first place.

Another problem with dieting is the conflicting information we hear about it. For example, for many years the American population was told that polyunsaturated fats would save lives and produce longevity. Now that relationship is not so clear. In fact, it has been suggested that certain types of cancer are actually *increased* by polyunsaturates. In the last few decades a large number of people switched from butter to margarine in order to benefit their cholesterol levels. But a study in the *New England Journal of Medicine* (Summer 1990) suggests that margarine not only increases cholesterol overall but actually reduces HDLs, the so-called good cholesterol. Some would have us believe that the answer to weight control lies in little packages of high-protein beverages. Others assert that the key can be found in the latest diet book. Should we eat more carbohydrates or fewer? No fish or only fish? There are dozens of examples of things we thought were good for us that have turned out to be damaging.

Perhaps the biggest distinction between our modern nutritional understanding of diet and that of Ayurveda is that modern nutrition analyzes food only in terms of its material qualities. Yet a biochemical approach to dieting ignores some very human issues: What about fulfillment? What about pleasure? What about the emotional and even spiritual benefits we experience from enjoying the foods we eat? The very idea of dieting suggests that these aspects of eating count for nothing, that the body will actually be better off when it's subjected to the *punishment* of severely restricted food intake.

The body responds to repression by rebelling—with massive sensations of hunger, with slowed metabolism, and even with disease. Diets that impose stress on your physiology by cutting off its natural inclinations invite this rebellion, which occurs at the level of every cell in your body.

Ayurveda is completely opposed to diets that ignore the needs of the entire mind/body system. Instead, we must return to the principle of balance. By understanding and heeding the needs of your body type, you can let your body tell you what your real hunger level is, when to eat, and what foods are best for you. This is the basis of a comprehensive diet that fulfills all the requirements of body, mind, and spirit.

So Ayurveda not only recognizes the material values of food but acknowledges that a more basic influence is exerted by everything we eat. This influence takes place at the connection between mind and body that we call intelligence. By calling our attention to this basic level of intelligence, Ayurveda reveals that the problem of overweight depends on the way food is processed in our physiology: How much of it is stored as fat rather than burned up as energy? If we eat in a way that produces energy rather than fat and ama, calorie-counting is no longer important.

KAPHA-REDUCING FOODS

In previous chapters, you learned that the dosha that governs the structure and maintains the stability of the physiology is Kapha. People who are overweight almost always have an imbalance of Kapha, perhaps accompanied by imbalances in the other doshas as well. The precise nutritional system of Ayurveda analyzes every factor in the environment, including every food, in terms of its influence on Vata, Pitta, and Kapha. Certain foods are known to reduce Kapha in the physiology. Eating these foods actually helps to transform your metabolism so that energy is produced instead of fat. Thus, making these foods part of your diet will help you reach and maintain your ideal weight without having to count calories or go on an uncomfortable diet. You should review and become familiar with the list below, but you should also understand that it is not something you need to follow rigorously. Simply try to include these foods in your diet as much as possible on a regular basis. And because they help to produce balance, you'll find that you will enjoy eating them.

FOODS THAT HELP REDUCE KAPHA

- Favor foods that are light, dry, and warm.
- Favor foods that are spicy, bitter, and astringent.
- Some specific recommendations:
- **Dairy.** Low-fat milk is better. It is best to boil the milk before you drink it—this makes it easier to digest. Let the milk cool, and drink

it when it is warm. (Cold milk will increase Kapha.) Do not drink milk with a full meal or with sour or salty food, as this makes it difficult to digest. You might add one or two pinches of turmeric or ginger to whole milk before boiling it, to further reduce the Kapha qualities in the milk.

- **Fruit.** Lighter fruits, such as apples and pears, are better. Pomegranates, cranberries, and persimmons are also good.
- **Sweeteners.** Honey is excellent for reducing Kapha.
- **Beans.** All beans are fine.
- **Grains.** Barley, corn, millet, buckwheat, and rye are best because they are light.
- **Spices.** All spices are good except salt, which increases Kapha.
- **Vegetables.** All vegetables are fine. The following vegetables are especially effective in reducing Kapha: radishes; asparagus; eggplant; green, leafy vegetables; beets; broccoli; potatoes; cabbage; carrots; cauliflower; pumpkin; lettuce; celery; sprouts.
- **Meat and fish** (for nonvegetarians). White meat from chicken or turkey is best. Fish is also fine.

PRACTICAL TECHNIQUES FOR RESTORING BALANCE

There are several powerful techniques that can help in reestablishing balance in a person who has become overweight. One of the most useful is the *liquefied diet.* I recommend following a liquefied diet one day each week. This will not only allow you to eat lightly on that day but will directly eliminate ama and strengthen digestion.

This liquefied diet is a very powerful addition to your routine. You should continue it once a week until you've lost all the weight that is appropriate for you. *Remember:* This is not a fast, nor is it necessary to buy liquefied protein solutions or anything of that sort. You may include any food you like as long as it is liquefied first. But because this is a purifying technique to eliminate ama, it's best to use foods that are fresh and wholesome.

Don't, for example, try to liquefy lasagna or pizza or meat. Soups, herbals teas, fresh fruit or vegetable juices, warm milk, and grains blended with water all work very well; with a few exceptions, you may take any item you like, add some warm liquid to it, and put it in your blender. You may take liquefied food or liquids as often as you like during the day. Some people find that they feel absolutely comfortable and energetic just taking fresh fruit juices. Others find that they need more substance in the diet, such as liquefied grains and vegetables. Follow the routine according to your level of comfort. When you use the liquefied diet properly, you should feel more energetic and light. However, if you are in the habit of jogging or performing other vigorous exercise, you might want to moderate that activity on the days you follow the liquefied diet.

The second technique I'd like to suggest is very effective for cleansing ama from the system. It is very simple, but it can be one of the strongest parts of an Ayurvedic weight control program. It involves nothing more than sipping hot water frequently throughout the day.

I mentioned earlier that ama is sticky. Just as you use hot water to wash dishes that are greasy or sticky, you can use hot water to dissolve ama gradually from your system. There is, however, a specific routine that you must follow to produce this effect.

First, the water must be very hot, so that you have to blow on it before you sip. If you have trouble with hot drinks, don't worry—you'll become accustomed to taking hot water within a few days. Second, the amount of hot water you drink is less important than how frequently you drink it. For best effect, the water should be sipped about every thirty minutes. If this is too frequent for you, take one or two sips of hot water at least once an hour. You can have much more of it if you like, but take at least one or two sips every thirty to sixty minutes. You may have other liquids during the day, but always take your hot water. After a few days, you'll feel so soothed and balanced from the hot water that you'll even begin to look forward it.

You may find yourself urinating more frequently during the first few weeks of the hot water program. This is because the body is beginning to flush itself out, to remove toxins and impurities from the system. It's a sign that something powerful is happening. After a few weeks, your urine will return to normal, but ama will continue to be dissolved from your system.

1. Begin using these two important techniques for eliminating ama. Adding them to your daily routine will greatly enhance your progress.
   - Once a week, eat a liquefied diet. Foods that you might include are soups, herbal teas, fresh fruit or vegetable juices, warm milk, or grains blended with water. You can liquefy any food in your blender, but remember to avoid eating foods that are not fresh or wholesome, as well as heavy foods such as lasagna, pizza, and meat.
   - Sip hot water frequently throughout the day. Remember that the water should be very hot and should be sipped often, about every half-hour. You might want to fill a thermos with hot water and keep it with you throughout the day.
2. Try these dietary suggestions to improve your digestion:
   - In general, meat increases Kapha and is more likely to produce ama than other foods. Favor chicken and fish over red meats, and try to keep several days a week completely meat-free.
   - Include plenty of fresh, cooked vegetables and grains.
   - Favor warm, light foods. Choose hot, cooked foods rather than cold foods (as hot foods are easier to digest and help balance the Kapha dosha).

- While cooked food is easier to digest and assimilate, you can include some raw vegetables and salads in your diet, according to taste. Raw fruits are also fine.
- Use fresh or powdered ginger in cooking to stimulate your digestion and eliminate ama. Other spices that stimulate digestion are cumin, turmeric, cardamom, cinnamon, clove, mustard seed, and black pepper.
- Try eating ginger just before your meal to stimulate your agni, or digestive fire.

EATING TO TRANSFORM YOURSELF

Here are some other dietary suggestions. By following them, you can transform your physiology from one that stores fat every time you eat to one that produces energy, vitality, and ojas.

- Favor chicken and fish over red meats, and try to have several days a week that are completely meat-free. Red meat increases Kapha and is more likely to produce ama than other foods.
- Try experimenting with recipes that use more freshly cooked vegetables and grains. You may want to try some new recipes that inspire you to emphasize these important nutritional elements. Be sure to include those vegetables and grains that are on the list of Kapha-reducing foods (page 68). Remember, the fresher the food, the more ojas it contains. Fresh fruits and vegetables are better than frozen, and frozen ones are better than canned.
- Pick hot food over cold at every meal. Eat a hot lunch instead of a sandwich, hot apple pie instead of ice cream, grilled fish instead of tuna salad.
- Ginger, a spice that is particularly good for reducing Kapha,

helps to stimulate digestion and eliminate ama. Try using fresh or powdered ginger in your cooking. Special preparations of ginger can be taken at the beginning of a meal to strengthen digestion so that the food is better assimilated.

- **Ginger Pickle.** Grate a small amount of fresh ginger root. Squeeze some fresh lemon juice on it and add a pinch of salt. Eat one or two pinches of ginger pickle (according to taste) a few minutes before your meal.
- **Ginger Juice.** Peel a 1-inch section of fresh ginger and cut it into slices. Using your blender, blend the ginger with ¼ cup of water to make a juice. Sweeten with honey, and drink a small amount (according to taste) a few minutes before your meal.
- **Ginger Tea.** If you don't have fresh ginger, try this method. Put a cup of water in a saucepan. Add a pinch of powdered ginger and bring to a boil. Let it cool slightly and take several sips a few minutes before your meal. You can gradually increase the amount of ginger, up to ⅛ teaspoon.

- Spices can make food more digestible and produce less ama. Particularly useful spices include cumin, turmeric, cardamom, cinnamon, cloves, mustard seeds, and black pepper. As these spices reduce Kapha, they increase the metabolic rate and help to convert food into energy instead of fat.
- Cutting back on sweets is difficult for many Kapha types, but you may find that a one-week trial on a low-sugar or sugar-free diet will give you more energy. This will also help you to deal with compulsive cravings for sweets. In chapter 7 you'll learn that the sweet taste derives not only from sugar but from foods such as bread and pasta. This taste is an essential part of everyone's diet, but it should be taken in moderation by those who wish to lose weight. Honey is the one sweet that actually

has the property of reducing Kapha, but you should note that Ayurveda says never to cook with or heat honey, as doing so will produce ama.

• Deep-fried foods of any kind will aggravate Kapha, so it's better not to eat them. However, it's not necessary to eliminate all fats. Almond, corn, safflower, and sunflower oils can all be included, and olive oil is also good.

• Restaurant food has to be carefully chosen by Kapha types. In general, it's hard to lose weight when you eat mostly in restaurants. The food is far too oily, salty, and sweet—the three tastes that increase Kapha. Despite recent findings on the high fat content of some Oriental cooking, this can still be a good choice in better restaurants, if you concentrate more on vegetables than on meat.

• Generally, Ayurveda prefers that all food be cooked, since that makes it easier to digest and assimilate. However, small amounts of raw vegetables and salads can tone the digestive canal. Just eat them according to your desire and taste. Fruits are fine to eat raw, of course.

• Soft drinks, especially low-calorie drinks, make up a significant part of many dieters' daily program. However, the carbonation actually disturbs the digestive process. It produces ama and distorts our natural sensations of hunger, giving rise to irregular and false signals. As much as possible, reduce or eliminate carbonated beverages from your diet. At first you may miss them, but within a few weeks you'll feel much better without them. Try substituting water or fresh juices.

• As much as possible, avoid packaged foods. Meals prepared from freshly cooked foods will be lively in nature's intelligence; packaged foods are generally old and lifeless—without Prana (life force), as Ayurveda would say. You may have noticed that nature herself packages foods, and each package contains a different aspect of nature's intelligence. Consider the yellow packaging of the banana, or the bright packaging of an orange, and how you find the delicious and unique qualities of nature's intelligence inside. These are the best kinds of packaged foods to include in your diet.

• Try to avoid strong stimulants such as caffeine and alcohol. Most people take these in an attempt to compensate for fatigue and imbalance, but they produce no beneficial effects. Over time, they exacerbate the symptoms they were supposed to correct.

• In many people, the satiety threshold, or level at which you feel satisfied from food, can be altered if you take in a sweet taste first. So if you start a meal with dessert, you may find that this by itself will alter the level at which you'll feel satisfied. Of course, if you've had dessert to begin your meal, don't eat it again at the end!

HERBAL SUPPLEMENTS FOR WEIGHT CONTROL

It's easy to get the idea that there's a pill to solve every problem. New drugs are constantly being developed for everything from headaches to heart disease, and these are aggressively marketed to physicians as well as to the public. It's no surprise, then, that there are shelves full of diet pills in every pharmacy, and most people who are struggling to lose weight go through a phase of trying to find a chemical solution to their problem. This may be profitable for the pharmaceutical industry, but it can be very destructive to the mental and physical health of the consumer.

Simply put: *Diet pills will not help you achieve your ideal weight.* Many of them are nothing more than diuretics, which produce an illusory weight loss by causing the body to eliminate fluids. Most people experience disturbing side effects from diuretics. All diet pills are much more likely to produce depression and anxiety than a long-term solution to the problem of overweight.

The Ayurvedic approach to drugs in general is quite different from what we're used to in the West. In fact, the herbal
preparations Ayurveda recommends cannot even be referred to
as drugs in the usual sense of the word. Most of the pills prescribed by Western physicians or sold over the counter in phar-
macies are artificially manufactured, highly concentrated
materials that the body treats as foreign substances. While
there's no doubt that commercially produced drugs are important in the treatment of many acute health problems, they are
not helpful for chronic conditions such as overweight that derive from the physiological constitution of the individual.
Herbal supplements, on the other hand, can be of great benefit in weight control, without the negative side effects of conventional drugs.

According to Ayurveda, herbs are really a link between the
body of a given individual and the larger environment of the
world, or even the universe. Herbs are essentially manifesta-
tions of *light*. Through the process of photosynthesis, radiant
energy of the sun is transformed into the physical object of a
plant. By ingesting the plant in the form of an herb, you are ac-
cessing the cosmic power of the universe in a very tangible way.
You are literally putting yourself in touch with the source of all
life. Whenever you make use of an herbal preparation, you
should be aware of this profound connection. Western medicine teaches us that if we simply put a tablet in our mouths,
without thinking about it, our health problems will disappear.
But Ayurveda recognizes that the act of taking any substance
into the body has much larger implications, which demand a
higher level of awareness on the part of the individual.

Although conventional drugs are usually classified according to their chemical composition or molecular structure,
Ayurvedic herbs are described in much less technical terms such
as their taste, their qualities of heat or cold, and their effects on
digestion. No one ascribes any importance to the taste of an as-

pirin tablet, and certainly not to that of a diet pill, but in fact the taste of any substance has a direct influence on the nervous system and the body as a whole, and has particular effects on each of the three doshas. In the same dosha-specific way, some herbs foster heat in the body, which increases Pitta and speeds digestion, while others are cooling and refreshing, which calms Pitta but strengthens Vata and Kapha. Clearly, these qualities directly influence the body's weight.

Ayurvedic herbal supplements are useful for weight control as part of an overall strategy that seeks to balance the individual at all levels—body, mind, and spirit. Although the constitution and the nutritional needs of each person are unique, certain combinations of herbs generally have proven useful in controlling weight. These combinations are available through Ayurvedic resources, the addresses of which are provided at the back of this book.

- **Haritaki,** which reduces accumulated Vata. Although overweight is usually a result of a Kapha imbalance, Vata dosha can also be the source of the difficulty when it accumulates as a result of blockages in the physiology. In addition to obesity, this can cause other problems of the digestive system such as bloating, gas, and constipation.
- **Amalaki,** which rejuvenates tissues, relieves irritations of the digestive system, and stabilizes blood-sugar irregularities that can manifest as unhealthy food cravings. In Sanskrit, *amalaki* means "nurse" or "mother"; this herb is one of the most powerful nurturing and healing agents in all of Ayurvedic medicine.
- **Bibihitaki,** which liquefies and expels Kapha accumulations in the digestive system. It is also useful as a strong but safe laxative.
- **Vidanga,** which is an important anti-ama element. It cleanses the digestive system of obstructions and prevents

symptoms such as bloating and heartburn. It is particularly useful for obesity caused by Pitta imbalance, which is characterized by ravenous appetite and a consequent tendency to overeat.

- **Katuka,** which is often prescribed for fevers but whose toxin-destroying properties are also useful in dissolving ama.
- **Brahmi,** which calms the nerves and mind. It is especially beneficial for dealing with the emotional causes of overeating, which typically appear as addictions to sugar and other forms of carbohydrates.
- **Guggul,** which reduces fat and toxins. Although it may increase appetite, the desire will be for healthful foods that are unlikely to exacerbate weight problems, and these cravings will replace those for high-fat or sugary foods.
- **Chitrak,** which reduces hyperacidity and promotes digestion. By increasing the efficiency with which foods are absorbed by the body, chitrak prevents stagnation in the digestive system and the accumulation of ama.

Herbal preparations are particularly well suited for reducing Kapha, which is the basis of many weight problems. Most herbs are of bitter, astringent, or pungent taste, and these are effective counters to the sweet cravings that often characterize Kapha imbalance. In any case, herbs are far more effective and less dangerous than any diet pills on the market.

THE EFFORTLESS DIET

For many readers, the dietary changes suggested in this chapter may seem too demanding at first. You should realize, however, that the ideas behind them are simply natural principles that you should have been following all along. These principles will bring about not only weight loss but all the qualities of health that ojas implies: a feeling of lightness in your body, ex-cellent energy, improved appetite, superior digestion, stronger resistance to disease, greater physical strength and stamina, and, most important, a sense of real happiness.

Once you begin to experience the benefits of this program, it will require no effort to continue. In fact, you won't be able to resist it. But if you find it's a strain to incorporate all of these things at once, select those that are most relevant to your life and your present situation and therefore are easiest for you. Later, based on your success, you can add those elements that you left out in the beginning.

6

Exercise Without Strain

Your body was designed for physical activity; the impulse to exercise is a natural human tendency. This can be seen very clearly in babies and children, who are constantly in motion, often just for the sheer joy of it. This joy in using the body can be retained throughout life. But if you don't presently feel that impulse, if you've become accustomed to a sedentary lifestyle, distance has come between you and nature. The cause of that distance is imbalance, which transforms natural vitality into fatigue and erodes motivation.

That imbalance does not have to be permanent. In this chapter you'll learn how to reawaken your body's inherent love of activity by following a few simple Ayurvedic principles—and you'll see remarkable benefits from doing so.

What is the purpose of physical exercise? Cherak, one of the first Ayurvedic physicians, said: "From physical exercise, one gets lightness, capacity to work, firmness, tolerance of difficulties, diminution of physical impurities, and strengthening of digestion and metabolism." But Cherak goes on to assert a classic Ayurvedic note of moderation. Although exercise is suitable for everyone, too much can be as damaging as too little.

In other words, just because something is good for you doesn't mean that more of it is better, and an effective exercise program must be based on the needs of the individual. The proper type and amount of exercise should be calculated to suit your individual needs. Excessive physical training can lead to higher incidence of hypertension, arthritis, and heart disease. Because of this, some countries in Eastern Europe have begun deconditioning programs for their Olympic athletes, who were not as healthy as the rest of the population. In this country, professional athletes do not live as long as the average American, who has a life expectancy in the late seventies. The life expectancy of a professional football player is somewhere in the late fifties. So there are definite risks associated with making an obsession of physical conditioning.

According to Ayurveda, exercise should produce energy, strength, and vitality, not use them up. If you feel exhausted and strained at any point in your workout, something is wrong.

CREATING A FAT-BURNING PHYSIOLOGY

Let's look in some detail at three of the most common errors people make regarding exercise.

• First, an individual may engage in only sporadic exercise, or none at all. Inactivity is very bad for your health. Studies have revealed significant differences between the recovery rates of hospital patients who were totally inactive, simply lying in bed all day, and those who performed even very small amounts of physical activity, such as standing up briefly or walking across their rooms. Of course, very few people outside of hospitals are completely sedentary. Yet many of us fail to get more than minimal physiological benefit from our everyday activities because these are performed in an unfocused, irregular manner.

The benefits of exercise derive more from frequency than from length or intensity of performance. This is an extremely important point. Walking or even running around the block once a week will have almost no effect on the physiology. But walking around the block once a day, interspersed with occasional longer walks, will produce measurable improvements in your metabolism, and this can have a major effect on your weight. Many people, conditioned to think in terms of calories, assume that a short, intense workout can help them to lose weight because they'll burn a large number of calories in a brief period of time. But the number of calories used in even the most intense exercise is insignificant in terms of weight loss. You would have to jog for hours to burn off the caloric content of just one steak dinner. Effective weight control isn't achieved through simplistic "calories per minute" ratios. The real key is to reconstitute your metabolism so that your body functions in a higher "gear" even when you're not exercising. This is achieved by regular exercise that challenges but doesn't strain your physiology.

• A second common error involves performing exercises that are unsuited to your particular physiology. Nature operates according to its own powerful logic, but the mechanics of this logic may not be exactly what you expect. For example, it might seem reasonable that an extremely overweight person should exercise very intensely, because the exertion should be in direct proportion to the size of the problem. But this is untrue. In reality, a very overweight person should perform *light exercise for long periods of time.* This is the only way the metabolism of such an individual will begin to burn fat. Studies show that short bursts of activity burn carbohydrates; it takes longer, ongoing exercise to burn fat. What's more, trying to exercise like a highly conditioned athlete is bound to be demoralizing for anyone who's extremely out of shape—and it will become even more demoralizing when the hoped-for results fail to materialize.

• The third common mistake is overexercising. By demanding too much of your body, you risk injuries ranging from sprained muscles to heart attacks. But beyond the possible physical consequences, overexercising creates the very sort of stress that you should be trying to avoid. Using your body should be a pleasurable activity. It should never become a chore. This is something that many goal-oriented, highly disciplined people find hard to understand, since the ethos of "no pain, no gain" may have served them well in their careers. Even the phrase *working out* implies that exercise should be hard and difficult. But Ayurveda suggests that physical benefits can't coexist with mental stress. Human beings are truly mind/body systems. What is beneficial for one part of the physiology can't be a strain on the other.

EXERCISE AND AYURVEDA

Many people feel that the entire relationship between exercise and weight control can be reduced to a simple equation comparing the number of calories consumed with the calories burned up through exercise and other activities. But programs based on these numbers have been unsuccessful in producing permanent weight loss. In addition, this type of analysis does not explain a commonly observed phenomenon: that certain overweight people who follow extremely restricted caloric diets still fail to lose significant weight. As we've discussed, the reason for this phenomenon is that our metabolisms begin to reset themselves in order to protect the physiology against starvation. So the less you eat, the slower your metabolism gets, and the more weight you gain.

When we begin to exercise, we give the body a new quantum mechanical signal that we are going to be active, energetic, vital people. We are telling ourselves that from now on we are going to begin to draw from available energy sources through our physical activity. Your physiology can then respond in a number of ways, depending on your body type and the kind of activity you're undertaking. Your body may begin to burn fat, which is what you want, or it may simply rely on blood sugar to fulfill the short-term energy requirement. By combining the correct physical activity with appropriate nutritional principles—which also signal our bodies at the quantum mechanical level—you can begin to reset your biological thermostat to a level where fat is more easily burned and food is converted into life-giving energy. This can dramatically change your experience of living. Many people feel transformed by regular exercise, not only in terms of their weight but in how they look and how they feel.

In Ayurveda, all of this is simply understanding and communicating with the doshas, and especially with Kapha dosha, which is usually responsible for overweight. Exercise, which is movement, has the property of reducing Kapha. But it's important to exercise properly so that in reducing Kapha we do not increase or disturb Vata by creating stress. Proper exercise, especially that which we refer to as *neuromuscular integration*, meets these requirements. Neuromuscular integration balances all three doshas at once. These exercises, which derive from the yoga tradition, not only provide physical benefits but also foster communication between mind and body.

Let me repeat: the thing to remember about exercise is that it doesn't have to be strenuous to be effective; and for most people, if it is strenuous, it may well be counterproductive. We are an extremely sports-conscious society. We're used to seeing athletes competing on television, starring in movies, or endorsing products in advertisements. But these overdeveloped individuals shouldn't be your role models for developing a personal exercise program.

Here are some practical guidelines for healthy exercise that are applicable to all body types:

• *In general, work to about 50 percent of your limit.* If you can swim twenty laps, swim only ten. If you can bicycle fifty miles, ride twenty-five. Our total capacity represents all the energy available at that time from our physiology. What we want is not to *expend* all of our energy but to *produce* more energy. So stop at about 50 percent. At that point you should still feel energetic and comfortable, never strained or tired. With regular exercise, your conditioning will improve and your total capacity will grow, so the 50 percent of that capacity will also increase.

• *Ayurveda recommends regular exercise, preferably seven days a week.* The reason many intensive exercise programs recommend three or four days of activity per week is that they use up all of the energy available to your physiology. They create stress and then allow rest for recuperation so that the process can begin again. But eventually the body breaks down or burns out, and the sequence is broken. Any exercise program that is inherently not enjoyable can never last long, no matter how many rest periods are built in. People simply won't do it if they don't enjoy it. *Remember*: by contrast to "no pain, no gain," the Ayurvedic principle is "no strain produces maximum gain."

• *Use your breathing and perspiration rates as indicators of exercise intensity.* In general, rapid breathing and heavy perspiration mean that you are straining your physiology. No exercise should be so challenging that you can't accomplish it while breathing through your nose. If you find you have to breathe through your mouth, either cut back on the intensity of your workout or switch to another activity. Pay attention to your breathing, which should be slow and deep. This is one of the best indicators of the effectiveness of any exercise.

Two excellent Ayurvedic exercises that focus on breathing are known as *bhastrika Pranayama* and *kapalabhati*. In the first of these activities, the abdominal muscles work like bellows, which is what bhastrika means in Sanskrit. All breathing is done through the nose only, so this technique should not be attempted if you have a cold or if for any reason your sinuses are congested. To begin, sit straight up on the floor or in a chair. Your arms should be parallel to your sides and bent upward at the elbows, with your hands in fists at approximately shoulder height. Once you've established the starting position, inhale and exhale a single deep breath through your nose. Then, as you take another deep breath, raise your arms straight up and, as they reach full extension, open your fists and extend your fingers. Now quickly lower your arms back to the starting position while simultaneously exhaling through your nose. Keep your hands facing forward throughout this exercise. Do this at a steady tempo of about one cycle per second. Continue for two or three sets of fifteen repetitions.

Kapalabhati is another breathing exercise that can activate the lungs and cardiovascular system to a level equivalent to that of jogging, a vigorous activity. The primary purpose of kapalabhati, however, is to cleanse metabolic wastes from the body. This is an extremely important benefit for individuals who are in the process of losing weight and whose metabolisms may not yet be working at high efficiency. Moreover, since kapalabhati accelerates the heart rate without requiring a great deal of exertion from the large muscle groups of the body, it is a particularly useful exercise for people who aren't at the high level of physical conditioning required by conventional athletics.

The technique consists of a series of short, powerful exhalations, each followed by a passive inhalation. To begin, sit with your back straight, either on the floor or in a chair. Your shoulders should be back, and your abdominal muscles should be free to move. Correct posture is extremely important in kapalabhati, because the abdominal muscles must be able to relax thoroughly when you inhale.

Once your posture is established, begin breathing through your nose to establish a rhythm of deep, even breaths. Then, just when you're about to exhale, contract your stomach muscles quickly and powerfully, which will force air out through your nostrils. This exhalation should be as complete as possible in one short, powerful blast.

Now, as you relax the muscles of your abdomen, inhalation occurs naturally. This should be completely passive, so avoid making any conscious effort to inhale. For the exercise to be effective, you must develop the ability to entirely relax your stomach muscles immediately after you inhale.

When you're first learning this exercise, try to exhale approximately once per second. Then gradually increase the rate to twice per second, but don't try to go any faster than that. As you become more adept, concentrate on exhaling as completely as possible and on relaxing your stomach muscles when you inhale. This is the essence of kapalabhati, and it is more important than the rapidity of your breathing.

You can use a mantra to increase the benefits of exercise. Research with instruments such as the electroencephalograph, or EEG, which measures electrical activity in the brain, has shown that certain mental states are beneficial to both physical and mental health. Specifically, researchers have found a very beneficial condition of "restful attention," which is typically observed during meditation. But restful attention can also be attained during exercise through the use of a mantra, or repeated pattern of sound. With your attention focused on your breathing, silently repeat the syllable *so* each time you inhale silently, and then, as you exhale, repeat the syllable *hum*. By using this mantra throughout your exercise period, you can enjoy the benefits of meditation and physical activity at the same time.

Remember that the best times to exercise are during the Kapha periods: 6:00 to 10:00 A.M. and 6:00 to 10:00 P.M. This is because the structure of your physiology is stronger and more tolerant at those times. The best exercises for weight loss meet two criteria: They involve continuous activity rather than starting and stopping, and they include motion by the large muscle groups in the lower half of the body, rather than just the arms. This kind of exercise is what the word *aerobic* refers to. Thus, although tennis and golf, for example, are great for relaxation, they do not fulfill the purposes of daily exercise.

By keeping these points in mind and making them part of your daily exercise program, you can gain enhanced clarity of thought, refined perception by all your senses, and lowered risk from many debilitating medical conditions such as hypertension and elevated cholesterol levels. But best of all, in terms of weight control, you can reconstitute your basal metabolic rate so that your body is burning fat all the time, not just when you're exercising. This kind of metabolism is characteristic of anyone who has made exercise a part of his or her daily routine. It's the fundamental difference between people who are truly "in shape" and those who follow a sedentary lifestyle.

DOSHA-SPECIFIC EXERCISES

In addition to the general principles outlined above, there are exercise guidelines that apply to the individual Ayurvedic body types.

Kapha types, for example, require the most exercise, Vatas require the least, and Pittas fall somewhere in between. If you are a two-dosha type, let your overall physical structure be your guide. If you're large, muscular, athletic, and Kapha is one of your dominant doshas, then put yourself in the Kapha category for the purpose of exercise. If your muscular and physical development is more modest, put yourself in the Vata category, which requires light exercise. Those in between should consider themselves in the Pitta category.

For Vata types, yoga, dance aerobics, short hikes, and light bicycling are the most suitable. Vata types should be cautious, however. Too much exercise can throw Vata out of balance. Activities suited to Pitta types are more vigorous, including skiing, walking or running, hiking, mountain climbing, and swimming. For Kapha types, running, weight training, aerobics, rowing, and dance are appropriate.

Of course, these are just a few examples of good exercises for each body type, and you shouldn't feel restricted to them. Above all, you should do something you enjoy. When people who do not enjoy exercise force themselves to do so, they release stress hormones such as cortisol, adrenaline, and noradrenaline, which may even have a detrimental effect on the immune system and other parts of the body. Also, if you dislike any particular form of exercise your body will resist it, and serious injury can result. On the other hand, if you enjoy a particular workout, your physiology will reflect that state of mind. Just playing with your children or flying a kite in the park can be more beneficial than a vigorous exercise program you don't enjoy.

However, if you don't get pleasure from exercise of any kind, it may be because you have a Kapha imbalance. As you regulate your Kapha dosha and bring it back into balance, you'll realize that in fact everyone enjoys some sort of exercise, and that excessive Kapha was responsible for making you feel dull and lethargic. Increase your activity very gradually in the beginning, following all the other recommendations you've learned about balancing Kapha. Then, as your level of activity becomes more vigorous, you'll begin to enjoy it.

All of these principles can be implemented through an activity such as walking, which is one of the most effective ways to satisfy your body's need for exercise. Although all body types respond well to walking, the ideal intensity and speed may vary from one dosha type to another: Kapha types may benefit from more vigorous, aerobic-type walking, while Vata types will respond better to a more leisurely, continuous stroll. A good daily walking routine would be thirty minutes in the morning and again in the evening. If your schedule doesn't allow this, try to do thirty minutes of brisk walking in the morning, or even three sessions of ten minutes each. Within a few days you'll begin to see a transformation.

Ayurveda also uses exercises from the yoga tradition, which are neuromuscular and neurorespiratory in their effect. This means they act not only on the muscular, cardiovascular, and metabolic systems but actually help to integrate mind and body as a unit to create perfect health. Instructions for these exercises appear below, and they make an excellent addition to your daily exercise program. These neuromuscular and neurorespiratory exercises can be performed in just fifteen minutes a day. You might do your thirty minutes of walking in the morning, for example, and then perform the neuromuscular and neurorespiratory integration exercises in the evening.

SUN SALUTE

The Sun Salute includes a series of twelve flexion and extension exercises that integrate the mind, body, and breath. The Sun Salute lubricates the joints, conditions the spine, and strengthens every major muscle group in the body. It creates balance, stability, suppleness, and flexibility.

General Guidelines for the Sun Salute

1. When you do the Sun Salute, allow a half-hour before a meal and three hours after a meal. If you practice other

meditation programs or yoga postures, the Sun Salute can be performed before them.

2. One cycle of the Sun Salute, consisting of twelve postures, is described below. Start with as many cycles as is comfortable, and gradually increase to a maximum of twelve. Do not strain. If you start to breathe heavily or begin perspiring, lie down and rest for a minute or two.

3. Hold each position for about five seconds. The Eight Limbs Position (position 6) is the only exception, as it is held only one second.

4. The Sun Salute uses a specific pattern of breathing—inhale or exhale—for each posture. You will be instructed to inhale during *extension* postures—because inhaling facilitates the extending and lengthening movements of the spine. You will be asked to exhale on the *flexion* postures, because this helps the body to fold, bend, and flex.

5. You'll see that there are two Equestrian positions per cycle. Use the same knee forward during the same cycle. Switch to the opposite knee for the next cycle, and continue alternating with each new cycle. Always do an even number of cycles so that both sides of your body are exercised in a balanced way.

6. Do not rush through the exercises; maximum value comes from doing them slowly. Each cycle takes one to two minutes.

7. After completing the final cycle, lie down on your back, arms at your sides, with palms facing upward, for two minutes. Just allow your attention to be easily on your body.

8. Be careful not to strain by stretching too far. The drawings show the ideal performance of each pose, but you should stretch only as far as your body is comfortable. Over time, more flexibility will develop. You should definitely not feel pain or discomfort while doing these

exercises. If even minimal performance of a particular posture causes discomfort, omit that posture. If you have back problems, consult your physician before starting these exercises.

How to Do One Cycle of the Sun Salute

1   SALUTATION POSITION

Start the Sun Salute with your feet parallel and your weight distributed evenly over your feet. Place your hands together, palms touching, at chest level. Breathe easily for about five seconds.

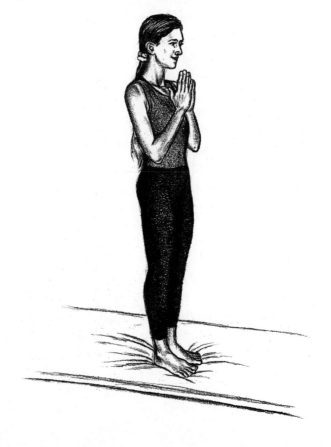

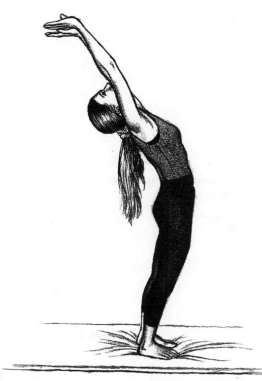

2 RAISED ARMS POSITION

As you inhale, lift your hands over your head, lengthening your spine easily in an extension posture.

3 HAND TO FOOT POSITION

As you exhale, bend your body forward and down into a flexion posture. Allow your knees to bend.

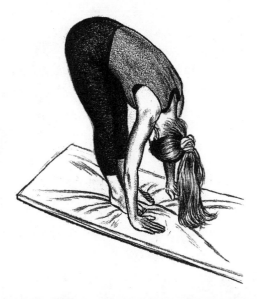

4   EQUESTRIAN POSITION

On the inhalation, extend your left leg back, knee to the ground. Allow your right leg to bend and your right foot to stay flat on the floor. Let your head and neck lengthen upward.

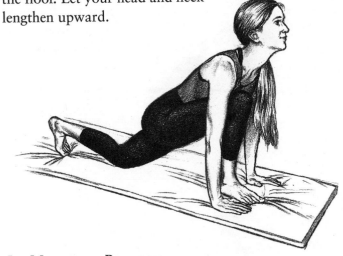

5   MOUNTAIN POSITION

As you exhale, place your right leg back, even with your left leg, pushing the buttocks up into a flexion posture. The body forms an even inverted V from your pelvis to your hands and from your pelvis to your heels.

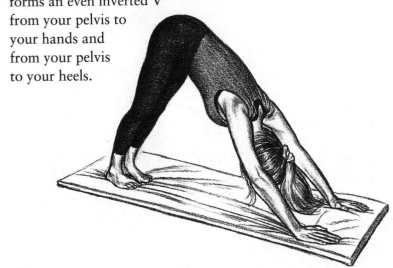

6   EIGHT LIMBS POSITION

Carefully drop both knees to the ground and allow your body to slide down at an angle, with your chest and chin briefly on the ground. Hold this for a second and then move smoothly into the next position.

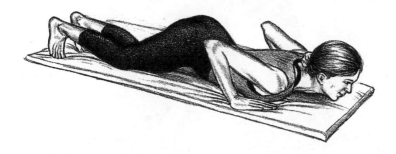

7   COBRA POSITION

As you inhale, lift your chest up and slightly forward while pressing down with your hands. Keep your elbows close to your body. Allow your spine to lift your head—do not start the movement with your head or lift your body with your neck.

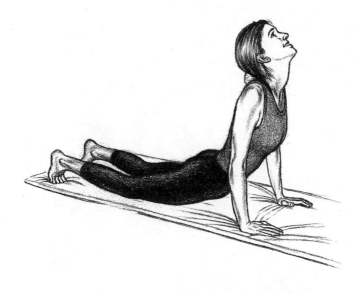

8   MOUNTAIN POSITION

While exhaling, raise your buttocks and hips in a flexion posture, the same as position 5.

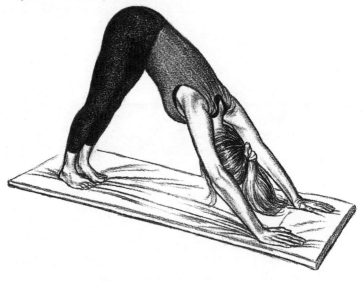

9   EQUESTRIAN POSITION

As you inhale, bring your right leg forward, between your hands, the same as position 4. Let your left leg extend backward, with the knee touching the ground. Your right knee will be bent and your right foot flat on the floor.

10 HAND TO FOOT POSITION

Repeat position 3. As you exhale, bend your body forward and down, coming down into a flexion posture. Allow your knees to bend.

11 RAISED ARMS POSITION

Repeat position 2. As you inhale, lift your hands over your head, lengthening your spine easily in an extension posture.

12 SALUTATION POSITION

Repeat position 1, ending the Sun Salute the same way you began, with your hands folded, palms together, in front of your chest. Breathe easily for about five seconds. Then begin the next cycle. (Position 12 becomes the first position for the second cycle; you can go directly into position 2 from here.)

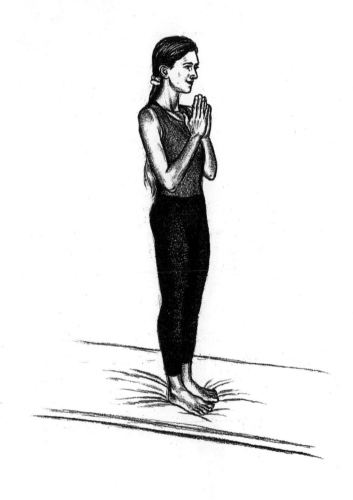

How to Do Pranayama

This simple neurorespiratory exercise, called Pranayama, creates balance throughout your body. It's ideal to do Pranayama after the neuromuscular integration exercises and before meditation.

1. Sit easily and comfortably with your spine as straight as possible.
2. Close your eyes and rest your **left** hand on your knees or thighs. For this exercise you will be using your thumb and the middle and ring fingers of your **right** hand.
3. Using your right thumb, close off your right nostril. Start by exhaling through your left nostril. Then inhale easily through your left nostril.
4. Now use your ring and middle fingers to close your left nostril. Exhale slowly through your right nostril, then easily inhale.
5. Continue alternating nostrils for about five minutes. Your breathing should be natural, not exaggerated. It may be a little slower and deeper than usual.
6. When you are finished, sit quietly with your eyes closed for a few minutes while breathing easily and normally.

Use the **Daily Ayurvedic Exercise Record** for the next two weeks to help you remember to exercise each day without strain.

DAILY AYURVEDIC EXERCISE RECORD

MONDAY

- Type of exercise _____

- Minutes spent exercising _____

- Describe how you felt before, during, and after exercising.
  (For example, you might feel exhilarated, energetic, or tired.)

  Before _____

  During _____

  After _____

TUESDAY

- Type of exercise _____

- Minutes spent exercising _____

- Describe how you felt before, during, and after exercising.
  (For example, you might feel exhilarated, energetic, or tired.)

  Before _____

  During _____

  After _____

WEDNESDAY

- Type of exercise _____

- Minutes spent exercising _____

- Describe how you felt before, during, and after exercising.
  (For example, you might feel exhilarated, energetic, or tired.)

  Before _____

  During _____

  After _____

DAILY AYURVEDIC EXERCISE RECORD

THURSDAY

• Type of exercise _____

• Minutes spent exercising _____

• Describe how you felt before, during, and after exercising.
  (For example, you might feel exhilarated, energetic, or tired.)

Before _____

During _____

After _____

FRIDAY

• Type of exercise _____

• Minutes spent exercising _____

• Describe how you felt before, during, and after exercising.
  (For example, you might feel exhilarated, energetic, or tired.)

Before _____

During _____

After _____

SATURDAY

• Type of exercise _____

• Minutes spent exercising _____

• Describe how you felt before, during, and after exercising.
  (For example, you might feel exhilarated, energetic, or tired.)

Before _____

During _____

After _____

DAILY AYURVEDIC EXERCISE RECORD

SUNDAY

- Type of exercise _____

- Minutes spent exercising _____

- Describe how you felt before, during, and after exercising.
  (For example, you might feel exhilarated, energetic, or tired.)

  Before _____

  During _____

  After _____

END-OF-THE-WEEK ASSESSMENT

Changes I've noticed in my mind or body since beginning to exercise.

_____

_____

_____

_____

_____

_____

_____

_____

_____

_____

_____

_____

7

OVERCOMING FOOD

CRAVINGS AND BINGES

For many people, the most challenging problem in any weight control program is dealing with food cravings, or so-called compulsive eating. Both of these difficulties can arise from following an improper diet over an extended period of time and from emotionally based self-destructive habits.

Eating improperly leads to food cravings because you don't feel satisfied at the end of a meal. No matter how much you eat, you still look in the refrigerator after the meal, thinking, "I'm not really hungry, but I still want something more." A similar tendency toward compulsive eating comes from old habits that are emotionally based. Since eating generates endorphins, which foster a sense of well-being, people often try to cover up their emotional concerns by eating. Unfortunately, they only add eating problems to whatever other problems they have.

In offering solutions, I want to acknowledge how difficult they can be for many people. While I think you'll find that Ayurveda has profound and effective solutions to these problems, I recognize that it will take time for new values to take hold in your life. My single most important suggestion is to be patient—not only with the program but with yourself. It's extremely damaging to criticize yourself each time you perceive that you've eaten in an unhealthy way. When you overeat, remember that it's because you're seeking to create more balance and greater satisfaction in your body and in your life. So self-criticism won't be helpful. Just follow the instructions below and gradually you'll be fulfilled in body, mind, and spirit.

THE IMPORTANCE OF TASTE

Ayurveda defines a balanced diet not just in terms of proteins, fats, carbohydrates, and so on, but in the context of another extremely important quality: *taste*. When your taste buds greet a bite of food, an enormous amount of information is delivered to your doshas. Trusting that your physiology knows how to use this information, Ayurveda allows you to eat a balanced diet naturally, guided by your instincts, and without turning nutrition into an intellectual headache.

Ayurveda recognizes six tastes: sweet, sour, salty, bitter, pungent, and astringent. You're no doubt familiar with the first four, but the other two may seem new. All spicy, hot-tasting food is pungent, while an astringent taste causes that dry puckering in your mouth, exemplified by pomegranates and beans.

Here are some examples of all six tastes:

- *Sweet* includes sugar, honey, rice, pasta, milk, cream, butter, wheat, and bread
- *Sour* includes lemons, cheese, yogurt, plums and other sour fruits, and vinegar
- *Salty* includes any food to which salt has been added
- *Pungent* includes chili peppers, cayenne, ginger, and any hot-tasting spice

- *Bitter* includes bitter greens, endive, chicory, romaine let-tuce, tonic water, spinach, and leafy greens
- *Astringent* includes beans, lentils, pomegranates, apples, pears, and cabbage

THE KEYS TO SATISFACTION IN EATING

Your body can perceive sweet taste in a dilution of 1 part to 200, salt in a dilution of 1 part to 400, sour in 2 parts to 130,000, and bitter in a dilution of 1 part to 2 million. This exquisite sensitivity has been developed by nature to allow food to speak to your doshas, to allow you to perceive directly what nature is trying to tell you about your needs. Significantly, research has shown that people who overeat have a high taste threshold, which means that their sensitivity to taste is less than that of those who don't overeat.

Taste can actually influence your metabolic rate. In fact, metabolism can be altered by as much as 25 percent through the use of various spices. So having a diet balanced in all six tastes is extremely helpful in satisfying food cravings, even those that have an emotional basis, because food has an effect not only on your physiology but on your psychological state, on the mind/body continuum. Taste directly influences emotions.

Consider all the expressions in the English language that refer to the senses. *Sweet,* for example, which increases the Kapha dosha, and Kapha is associated with the qualities of a sweet nature. We all use expressions like *sweet love* and *sweet babies* and *sweet memories.*

But that same sweetness can become cloying and possessive and greedy when there's imbalance of the doshas, and that imbalance is aggravated by eating too many sweet foods. Similarly, sour in excess produces resentment and envy—as in *sour grapes*—while in normal amounts it produces exhilaration. While a proper amount of bitter taste produces a bracing alertness, excessive bitter produces a lack of satisfaction in life. Grief, which makes life seem completely without satisfaction, is bitter. In this way, each of the six tastes can be described by its emotional connotations as well as its physical sensations.

IDEAS FOR PUTTING THE TASTES TO USE

Try to include foods from all six tastes in your diet on a regular basis. This will require some experimenting with different foods and new spices. If it's impossible to build all six tastes into every meal, at least experience each of them every day.

If you feel that your taste buds are not fully alert and receptive, try swishing a tablespoon of warm sesame oil in your mouth. Do this each morning and then rinse with warm water. Sesame oil has the quality of enlivening the taste buds and making them more discriminating and sensitive.

Of all the tastes, sweet is the one most often craved. Perhaps this is because sweetness has the most settling effect, and because it increases Kapha more than any other taste. If you crave sweets, make sure that your diet is thoroughly balanced: It should include all six tastes, and they should be served in a fresh, wholesome, nutritious, and balanced way. One food that Ayurveda recommends specifically to help heal cravings for sweets is milk. Milk itself is sweet, and it also has an extremely settling quality for the physiology. If you constantly long for sweets, try taking a cup of warm milk each day, perhaps as part of your breakfast.

Honey can also help with cravings for sweets. Honey is the only sweetener that actually has the property of reducing Kapha. Try taking lemon and honey water on a daily basis. This will help not only to satisfy your craving for sweets but to dissolve ama from your system. You may find that this makes an ideal beverage at breakfast. Honey can also be taken plain dur-

Write down foods and spices that you enjoy for each of the six tastes. Then plan a few meals that include all six tastes. Record how you felt after eating each meal.

BITTER

1.

2.

3.

4.

5.

6.

ASTRINGENT

1.

2.

3.

4.

5.

6.

PUNGENT

1.

2.

3.

4.

5.

6.

SWEET

1.

2.

3.

4.

5.

6.

SOUR

1.

2.

3.

4.

5.

6.

SALTY

1.

2.

3.

4.

5.

6.

MEAL PLANS USING ALL SIX TASTES

MEAL ONE

MEAL TWO

MEAL THREE

How did you feel after eating these meals? Did you feel more satisfied than usual? Write your experiences here.

MEAL ONE

MEAL TWO

MEAL THREE

ing the day in limited quantities, perhaps half a teaspoon three or four times a day.

Remember that herbs are an extremely important part of the Ayurvedic approach to health. Herbs, like all foods, influence the physiology on the basic level of nature's intelligence, but herbs can be used more precisely to influence a particular aspect of Vata, Pitta, or Kapha, or even other elements of your physiology. Review the list of herbs that can benefit weight control (page 73). Information for ordering specially prepared combinations of these herbs can be found at the end of this book.

BREATHING AWARENESS MEDITATION

Meditation is an extremely effective technique for dealing with emotionally based cravings and binges. Some concentration is required to make use of the method I'm about to introduce, but the rewards will certainly justify the effort. The inner peace you create through meditation can be the key to creating balance in your diet and all other daily activities.

Most of what goes through our minds is nothing more than habit. This constant background static of mental activity can take control of what you eat and of everything else in your life. But through meditation you can reach and take advantage of the healing silence that exists in the physiology when it's relaxed.

Please do not use this relaxation exercise while driving a car or operating any sort of machinery. Wait until you have some quiet time alone. Then, when you're ready to begin, sit quietly, holding your hands lightly at your sides or in your lap. Your eyes should be closed. Start to breathe lightly and easily, letting your attention follow your breathing. Feel the breath flowing down into your lungs. There's no need to inhale deeply or to hold your breath, just breathe normally. When you exhale, let your attention follow the air up out of the lungs and softly out through the nostrils.

Don't force any of this. Let your breath move gently and easily, with your attention following. Then make your breathing a little lighter. Again, don't force—just let it happen by itself. Continue this relaxed breathing for about five minutes, with your eyes closed and your mind focused on the easy, natural flow of your breath.

Just by paying attention to your breathing in this manner you can access a level of relaxation that will benefit every area of your life. As you gain experience in this technique, mental static will begin to disappear and so will the self-destructive eating behaviors that accompany it.

CONTROLLING EMOTIONALLY BASED EATING

To conclude this chapter, I want to present an idea you can use whenever you're having difficulty with emotionally based eating. In the long run, balancing the doshas through proper diet provides the most permanent solution, but this technique is useful until you have permanently solved the problem.

Whenever you think that you may be eating compulsively, ask yourself: "Is it food that I want or is there an emotional discomfort that I'm trying to satisfy by eating?" Remember, eating when you're not hungry will never satisfy the emotional need on a lasting basis, and will only produce further discomfort through the production of ama and increased fat.

Snacking is an impulse that arises from lack of satisfaction in your overall diet. Unfortunately, ama is produced by most snack foods. In order to end the snacking habit, review chapter 5, which describes how you can create satisfaction through a balanced diet. And remember that when you take lunch as the main meal and incorporate all six tastes, that dissatisfied feeling that leads to snacking will spontaneously dissipate.

There's an interesting basis for the phenomenon of late-night snacking. The second Pitta period of the day—from 10:00 P.M. to 2:00 A.M.—is not really intended for taking meals. Rather, it's a time when the body should use its metabolic processes to purify itself and digest any food remaining in the system. This is why it is not uncommon to wake up hot and sweaty between 10:00 P.M. and 2:00 A.M., especially if you've eaten a large dinner. But if you've stayed up and have remained active past 10:00 or 10:30, which are the optimum times for going to bed, you may feel hungry around midnight—and it will be hard to resist, because it is a natural impulse. However, this natural impulse has arisen only because you've allowed yourself to break from nature's underlying rhythms.

The key to defeating emotionally based or impulsive eating, then, is to balance your biological rhythms throughout the day. And always be aware of your hunger level. Whenever you feel the urge to snack, put your hand over your stomach and ask yourself: "What's my hunger level right now?" Experience the sensation fully, maybe even close your eyes. Perhaps you'll find the sensation is really calling for something else, and not for eating at all. Perhaps it's a sense of emotional discomfort that arises from something unsettled in your life. As you direct your attention to the sensation itself, many times that craving will dissipate and you will no longer need to snack.

If you close your eyes and sit quietly for twenty or thirty seconds, you'll usually be able to sense some physical sensation associated with the emotional discomfort you're experiencing. This physical sensation may be in the area of the heart, the stomach, or elsewhere. Now, while keeping your eyes closed, simply allow yourself to experience that physical sensation for a few seconds. Don't try to dissolve it, just experience it. Within a minute or two the physical sensation will usually begin to lessen or even disappear. And when you open your eyes, you'll find that the emotional pain you were experiencing has diminished. If you still feel hungry for food, then go ahead and eat. But many times the urge will have left you.

In all the Ayurvedic techniques you've learned, the objective has been to amplify and unfold the spontaneous, self-referral healing responses that are present in your physiology at all times. The perfect response to every situation as it occurs is *already* built into your system. You need not go anywhere to learn it, because it's already present within you: the ideal body, the perfect weight, the precisely balanced physiology.

Several years ago I had a patient who had tried every available diet and weight loss technique, but who still remained some fifty pounds above her ideal weight. There were periods, of course, when her weight went down, but the familiar pattern always reasserted itself. Within a few months the weight returned, faster than before.

In talking with this patient, it became clear that she had been casting about among all the dozens of weight control methods and had become confused and discouraged by their contradictory advice. So I began by asking her to do just one simple thing: For the next five days she should carry a thermos of hot water flavored with ginger, from which she should take a small drink several times each hour. Aside from the cleansing effects this would have on her physiology, I knew there would also be a number of important psychological benefits. The process of sipping the water on a regular schedule would consistently focus her attention on what was happening to her body. After a day or so, she would become aware of toxins beginning to emerge through symptoms such as the coating on her tongue. And then, after another few days, when these symptoms disappeared, she would realize that her unhealthy food cravings had disappeared along with them. This is exactly what happened.

I then suggested an additional technique: I asked my patient to begin carrying a small notebook. Whenever she was about to begin a meal, she would jot down her hunger level, using the Satisfaction Meter described in chapter 1. Then, when the meal was finished, she would again note her hunger level. Like the hot water, this procedure had benefits for both the body and the mind. Having to write down her hunger levels helped prevent overeating, and it also continued to focus her attention on her eating behavior so that she began to experience a sense of control. Instead of feeling that eating was something that just happened to her, she realized that it was something she could choose to do or not to do. It's important to realize that at no point was anything said about calories or fat content or avoiding certain foods. There was no need for any of that. Once her attention was focused, and once she began to experience the benefits of healthier eating habits, she naturally began to avoid self-destructive behaviors. And her weight began to go down.

Over the next few weeks I introduced her to the Breathing Awareness Meditation. I also suggested that she begin including all six tastes in her meals, and that she begin following a Kapha-pacifying diet and supplement this with the herbs mentioned in chapter 5. By this time she was feeling so much better that she began a program of regular exercise entirely on her own. It happened naturally, without any directives from me and without any sense of stress or strain on her part.

What was the result? My patient lost weight and kept it off, of course, but this was only part of a much larger transformation. Her whole experience of living changed, *and it was simply the result of using the very techniques I've presented in this book.*

No matter what's happened to you in the past, there's no reason why you can't achieve the same results as my patient, who had been disappointed so often. In short, you really can be slim effortlessly, and you can start today. It won't be drudgery, it will be an adventure.

There's a great poem by T.S. Eliot that says, in effect, we shall not cease from exploration, and the end of our exploring will be to arrive where we started and to know the place for the first time. Your health, and your life, is a journey that doesn't require you to go anywhere. It's a journey without distance, because deep inside you there is a god in embryo, and it has only one desire. It wants to be born.

Appendix:

How the Body Acquires, Uses, and Stores Energy

The human body is such a complex and unique creation that any metaphor for describing it is bound to be inadequate. But as a first step toward understanding how energy is obtained and utilized, it's helpful to think of the body as a kind of rechargeable battery. Like a battery, the human physiology receives energy from an outside source, which it then either stores in the form of fat and muscle or uses to satisfy a variety of needs. Solving a crossword puzzle, running after a bus, hammering a nail, or drinking a glass of water all require energy that originates somewhere outside the body, which is then used to accomplish these external tasks. At any given moment, however, a significant percentage of the fuel available to the body is required simply to maintain the *internal* processes of life. In Western medicine, this form of energy utilization is referred to as metabolism. More specifically, the term *basal metabolism* refers to the number of calories burned in a given time by a body at rest in order to sustain respiration, circulation, digestion, and other vital functions.

At this point, the battery metaphor begins to break down. A battery, after all, doesn't need any of its electricity just to remain a battery, but your body's metabolism has intrinsic energy requirements that must be met, or death will result. In the Ayurvedic view all of this is more than simply a collection of physical and chemical processes. *Consciousness* and *awareness* are important components in determining every aspect of how your body expends energy, and they're equally important in determining how the body gathers energy in the first place. Indeed, Ayurveda sees consciousness and awareness as essential elements of energy itself.

When you plug a battery into an electric socket and allow it to recharge, there's no mystery about where the energy comes from. It passes from the wires in the wall into the storage cell of the battery. Similarly, if you're feeling weak and run-down, but feel stronger after eating a nutritious meal, the cause-and-effect sequence is easy to recognize. But once again, the analogy is useful only up to a point. It would be very surprising, for example, if a battery were to regain its charge without being plugged into a socket. Yet there are many animals, and even significant numbers of people, who are able to sustain themselves on little or no food at all. A chameleon lying on a rock absorbs heat and light from the sun, which can continue its life even if it fails to find food. A frog half-submerged on a lily pad literally "drinks" through its skin, and can be poisoned by polluted water even if none ever enters its mouth. And there are many cases, some of them very well documented, of individuals from a variety of religious traditions who have lived for months or years virtually without food as we normally use the word.

This remarkable process can work in reverse as well. Hospitalized patients, who are often for good reason depressed, frequently derive little benefit from the bland meals they're offered, in spite of the fact that the food fulfills every "nutritional requirement" stipulated on a government chart. Family members who smuggle prohibited foods to these patients might be condemned from a conventional medical point of view, but it could be argued that conventional medicine has a very narrow idea of what a human being's nutritional requirements really include.

Let me be very clear, then, about the Ayurvedic view of nutritional energy: *what* it is, *where* it comes from, and *how* best to use it.

According to Ayurveda, there is one source of all energy, whether it's manifested in food or in sunlight or in the waters of the ocean. This single source is Prana, the life force that is active not only in every physical event, but in every thought and emotion as well. At present, Western technology accords no recognition to this fundamental energy, although it is a basic concept of Chinese medicine, where it is known as *Chi,* and is recognized by many other traditions as well.

Prana is easier to recognize in its effects than it is to define precisely, and it cannot be quantified in terms of calories or volts of electricity. But the reality of Prana is experienced whenever you feel truly *alive,* whenever your mind is clear and alert and your body is healthy and full of vitality. Ayurveda understands Prana as the foundation of good nutrition and a healthy metabolism, and of much more as well.

But this can easily give rise to an all too common misunderstanding: that is, that nutrition in anything but the narrowest sense is exclusively or even primarily a function of *eating.* In contrast, Ayurveda teaches that Prana can and should be acquired in a variety of ways. This has important implications for the entire topic of weight control, because when life-sustaining nutritional benefits are received from sources other than food, the need to eat diminishes. Or, putting it more simply, when you acquire Prana by other means, you'll be less dependent on eating—not only for nutrition, but also for the emotional satisfaction that is often mistakenly sought in food.

The notion of balanced breathing, for example, receives virtually no attention in the West, yet Ayurveda considers breath to be the most significant of all the body's functions. Breath is the physiology's main source of Prana, and the character of an individual's breathing also influences other vital activities, which are in turn sources of Prana themselves. Thoughts and emotions are directly linked to the pace and depth of your breathing, as are heart rate and production of hormones. What's more, deep breathing burns calories in very large numbers, so even in conventional Western terms an individual's style of breathing deserves recognition as a significant physiological variable. Yet most people never think of focusing attention on their breathing as a way of benefiting their metabolism, let alone as a means of putting themselves in touch with the life force itself.

It's important to remember that Prana is not a physical or tangible substance that can be held in the hand or looked at under a microscope. It can't be seen in a horse or a chair or a beautifully cut diamond. Yet, really, it can be "seen" in all of them, in everything, because Prana is manifest throughout the universe. It's present in every thought and feeling as well.

Christ said, "Man does not live by bread alone," and I understand this as an affirmation of the idea that nutrition has a spiritual dimension that simply must be recognized. To achieve health in any genuine sense, your body needs the life force of Prana every bit as much as it needs calories of protein or carbohydrates.

What are the implications of this for your everyday life, especially with regard to weight control? I have several suggestions that are unrelated to food, but one point specifically related to eating needs to be made. Elsewhere in this book we've discussed the importance of fresh food, properly seasoned and prepared, but let me once again emphasize the significance of eating with attention and intention. The physical or organic qualities of *what* you're eating can't be separated from *how* you're eating in an emotional and spiritual context. In a fast-paced, fast food culture, it may seem far-fetched to suggest that eating should be a spiritual activity. But that is exactly what I am suggesting if you are to nourish yourself with the Prana in food.

There's really nothing complicated about this. Simply *looking* at your food with focused attention—smelling the aroma of it, then tasting it with full awareness—will activate the Prana within you. And, very significantly for weight control, it has been shown that conscious awareness while eating elevates the metabolism, in some cases even to the point where even more energy is expended in consuming the meal than was present in the food itself. Yet the life force is increased rather than diminished, because a state of conscious awareness and positive emotion influences not only the measurable metabolic rate, but also the biological pathways through which the metabolized energy is used.

Dramatic evidence of this emerged during a study of cholesterol in rabbits. In order to study the origins of cardiovascular disease, several groups of rabbits were fed meals designed to elevate their cholesterol. The investigators expected the rabbits to develop hardening of the arteries, which is what happened to most of them, but one group of animals seemed relatively immune. Although identical food was being offered to all of the subjects, this single group of rabbits failed to develop the physical problems that appeared in the others. The experimenters were puzzled, until an unanticipated variable in the procedure revealed itself. The laboratory assistant who had been feeding the atypical group had stroked and cuddled them while they ate. The sense of peace and security this treatment evoked in the rabbits overcame the effects of a diet specifically designed to make them ill. So, the conclusion is obvious: the food you eat is important, but your feelings and your level of conscious awareness as you're eating it can be even more significant.

Now, quite apart from food or eating, here are some other important sources of Prana and some ideas for bringing their benefits into your life:

• *Recognize the importance of the air around you.* I've mentioned the benefits of controlled breathing, but the significance of *what* is being breathed should be emphasized as well. You can literally feel the truth of this with your own lungs. Think of how it feels to inhale the fresh air of a pine forest compared, for instance, to the exhaust-filled atmosphere of a big-city street. In the forest setting, the body automatically breathes more slowly and deeply, while in a traffic jam the breath reflexively becomes rapid and shallow, if only out of an unconscious instinct for self-preservation. Of course, the physical characteristics of the breathing are reflected in the thoughts that pass through your mind as well.

To enhance the Prana you acquire from the air around you, try to put yourself in touch with plants and vegetation as often as possible. With a little attention, this can be accomplished even by urban dwellers. Houseplants can transform the atmosphere as well as the decor of an office or apartment, and cities like New York and Chicago have botanical gardens that deserve regular visits. You'll find that the experience of actually being in a lush, green environment for a substantial time has benefits that endure long after you've departed.

• *Get in touch with the soil.* I mean this quite literally. You should make an effort to actually feel the ground every day. For thousands of years of human history, people were constantly in touch with the life-giving dirt beneath their feet, yet in today's concrete and steel environments one can actually pass a lifetime without ever coming in contact with the soil.

If you live in an area where it's at all possible to do so, I urge you to walk barefoot for a period of time each day. Even if you live in a city and there's only a tiny patch of unpaved ground beside your bus stop or the entrance to your apartment building, bend down and touch it. Put your attention on the Prana that's always present in that patch of ground. If you have the intention to feel it you *will* feel it, because it's there in every atom and every molecule, whether overgrown with summer weeds or buried under snow and ice.

• *Feel the warmth of the sun.* The sun is ultimately the source of all life, and the truth of this will be intuitively recognized by anyone who has seriously given thought to it. Life, which began in the light and warmth of the sun's rays, was celebrated in the sun-worshipping religions of virtually all ancient peoples. Regard for the achievements of modern science, or respect for contemporary religions, is not diminished by acknowledging the obvious core of truth in the beliefs of the past. By feeling the heat of the sun upon your skin, you are putting yourself in direct contact with the most powerful source of Prana that can be experienced on Earth. Of course, as you would with fire in any form, be respectful of the power of this energy and don't expose yourself to "too much of a good thing."

• *Regularly view the ocean or another large, natural body of water in your area.* If at all possible, allow the water to flow over you, or at least over your hands or feet. If your contact with water is largely limited to what comes out of a faucet, the difference in the feel of an uncontrolled, unregulated currently or tide will be instantly apparent. That difference, in a word, is Prana. It's the same difference that exists between mass-produced, denatured food and freshly harvested produce, or between the dead, icy draft of an air conditioner and a cool mountain breeze. It's a difference you'll come to recognize more and more by putting yourself in touch with the sources of Prana that once were worshipped, but that today are all too often ignored.

Finally, let me state what must be obvious by now. Just as all Prana is essentially the same, so all the sources of Prana are essentially one. The vapor that rises from the oceans to form the rain, the rain that falls to Earth to moisten the soil, and the sun that draws forth the crops are a single, holistic system. By putting yourself in direct contact with the elements of this system as I've suggested, you can enlarge the presence of the life force throughout your being. You can strengthen the Prana in your body and magnify the love in your soul.

Sources

More information on Mind/Body and Ayurvedic treatments, products, herbs, and educational programs can be obtained from the following organizations:

Quantum Publications
P.O. Box 598
South Lancaster, MA 01561
800-858-1808

Quantum Publications, Inc., is a Massachusetts corporation beneficially owned by Dr. Deepak Chopra and his family.

Sharp Institute for Human Potential and Mind/Body Medicine
8010 Frost Street, Suite 300
San Diego, CA 92123
800-82-SHARP

Ayurvedic Institute
1311 Menaul N.E., Suite A
Albuquerque, NM 87112
505-291-9698

American Institute of Vedic Studies
P.O. Box 8357
Santa Fe, NM 87504

American School of Ayurvedic Sciences
10025 NE 4th Street
Bellevue, WA 98004
206-453-8022

Maharishi Ayurved Products
P.O. Box 541
Lancaster, MA 01523
800-255-8332

Shivani Ayurvedic Personal Care Products
P.O. Box 377
Lancaster, MA 01523
800-237-8221

Auromere Ayurvedic Imports
1291 Weber St.
Pomona, CA 91768
909-629-0108

Deepak Chopra, M.D., is Executive Director of the Sharp Institute for Human Potential and Mind/Body Medicine in San Diego, California. The institute offers mind/body and Ayurvedic therapies in outpatient and residential settings in association with the Center for Mind/Body Medicine; training in mind/body and Ayurvedic medicine for health professionals and the general public; and research to validate the effectiveness of mind/body treatments. For further information, please call 1-800-82-SHARP.

INDEX